Practical Care of Sick Children

A manual for use in small tropical hospitals

**Pauline Dean and
G.J. Ebrahim**

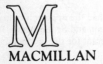

MACMILLAN

First published 1986
Reprinted 1990, 1991, 1992, 1994

Published by THE MACMILLAN PRESS LTD
London and Basingstoke
*Associated companies and representatives in Accra,
Auckland, Delhi, Dublin, Gaborone, Hamburg, Harare,
Hong Kong, Kuala Lumpur, Lagos, Manzini, Melbourne,
Mexico City, Nairobi, New York, Singapore, Tokyo*

ISBN 0–333–42347–X

Printed in China

A catalogue record for this book is available from
the British Library.

Acknowledgements
The authors are grateful to the following
- Dr Maureen Duggan and Professor David Morley who made many useful comments
  on the text.
- Sr. Una ni Riain and Miss Irene Morrison who gave valuable suggestions on the
  section dealing with designing and running a children's ward, based on their
  extensive experience of working in hospitals in Africa.
- Dr. F. Miller for his valuable comments and help on the chapter on Tuberculosis.
- Mr. R. L. Huckstep who kindly gave permission to use illustrations from his book
  'Poliomyelitis – a guide for developing countries'.
- The World Health Organisation for use of material on diarrhoea.
- Sr. N. Muldoon for help with the art work.
- The Ward Sisters and Nurses with whom the authors have had the opportunity to
  work, in particular Sr. Catherine Onyeugo, Sr. Victoria Simon and Sr. Soskenna.
- MISEREOR who have been most generous in providing a grant for the production
  of this book, for which we are most grateful.

Contents

Introduction

This book had its origin in a small mission hospital in Nigeria. Seventy four per cent of all paediatric admissions to the hospital were for nine preventable illnesses and other largely preventable conditions. The largest section of the book deals with these conditions, though some are given less space than the others. This is not because they are less important but because others have studied them well, written about them well, and the treatment is better known and carried out.

In all developing countries all hospitals outside the capital and the regional centres tend to be small, with far from ideal facilities or equipment, and chronically short of staff. There may be a small children's ward, but often the practice is to accommodate children with adults in a general ward. Those assigned to caring for sick children in such hospitals may not have had any paediatric training. The book is addressed to these colleagues who are faced with the impossible burden of dealing with large patient numbers with inadequate staff, unsatisfactory buildings and poor laboratory and other technical support. The hospital administration may have a somewhat vague policy or plan. It is our belief that if those of us who care for sick children in hospital took time regularly to consider the aims of the service and to discuss what is possible with limited personnel and funds, the standard of care can be considerably improved.

Hospitals and other health institutions in most national health services suffer from a rapid turnover of staff. Before a new arrival has properly settled in it is time to move again. There is hardly any opportunity for instituting change. In that respect we have been fortunate. One of us was resident in the mission hospital for many years. The hospital had a School of Nursing and therefore student nurses. We appreciate that the methods of working elsewhere may be different, and the hospitals may be staffed only by a handful of staff nurses and auxiliaries. But the principle is the same everywhere, viz the need for the staff of each ward to meet regularly and decide what they want to do, who is going to do it, and how it is to be done. The book was originally intended for nurses coming newly to work with sick children in a hospital in tropical Africa. It was intended for both trained nurses who may have been out of contact with sick children for some time and may wish to refresh their knowledge, as well as for newcomers like student nurses. We then decided to expand its scope to include physicians who may have had little or no paediatric training but who find themselves assigned to a children's ward with very little to fall back on.

We are fully aware that the book may not answer all the needs of those health workers who are involved in the day to day care of sick children in small tropical hospitals. Perhaps it may help if we state that much of the text came to be written following ward staff meetings. In another hospital, in a different locality and culture, the results may have been very different. The book is only an example for one hospital. It will be far more effective for the existing staff of any hospital to give time for meetings and discussions either to improve upon the book, or preferably even write their own manual.

● CHAPTER 1

History Taking

Good records are essential but paper may be in short supply. Keep as concise as possible but with essential facts. At the end make a list of the problems with which the child is presenting and any additional ones you think he has.

Complaint

It may be brief and exact, e.g. 'Loose stools and vomiting for 3 days'.
● In such a case get more precise details.
− How many stools in 24 hours?
− What do they look like?
− How many times did he vomit in 24 hours?
− Does anything start off the vomiting, e.g. coughing?
● **Always ask** 'So what medicine did the child receive for this?' Remember to enquire about home remedies or medicines from the traditional medicine man.
● Next ask 'Is there anything else?'

History may be long-winded and confusing. Parents may wish to describe not only the symptoms but also what in their opinion is causing them. Some such explanations may appear bizarre from the point of view of Western medicine. Ask the following questions.
● 'When was the child last quite well?'
● 'What was the first thing you noticed wrong?'
● 'What happened next?'
● 'What did you do?'
● 'And the next day?' − and go on until the days or weeks are covered.

1

Previous illnesses

- Ask what illnesses the child has had.
- If mother says *none*, ask specifically about measles, whooping cough and diarrhoea. Ever in hospital?

Child's background

With practice, this can be obtained fairly rapidly.
- What place in the family?
- Delivery: Normal? Feeding as a baby — breast fed? For how many months?
- Diet: When started solid foods? Which ones?

Present diet	Ask specifically how many times/week
a.m.	meat . . . ./wk
noon	fish . . . ./wk
p.m.	eggs . . . ./wk
	beans . . . ./wk
	groundnuts . . . ./wk

- Development: Sat up at ? months. Stood up? Walked? Talked?
- Immunisations and vaccinations?
- If school age, going to school?

Family and social history

- Father: Well? Work? Does it separate him from the family?
- Mother: Well? Living with father? Only wife?
- If other children: First child in family — alive or dead? If died, what age and what cause? Second child, and so on down through all the children.
- Any family sicknesses, e.g. TB?
- If parents are separated, who supports the mother?
- If father dead, who supports the mother?
- If child is brought by someone other than parents, why?
- Where do they live: Village? Town? Bush?

Specific complaints

● If loose stools
- Always ask how many a day?
- For how many days?
- What do they look like?   any blood or mucus?
- Any vomiting?   How many times a day?
- Has the child passed urine in the last 6 hours?
● If vomiting
- How many times a day?
- What makes child vomit?   coughing?   or after medicines? or just spontaneous?
- Any fevers?
● If cough
- What kind of cough? wheezy? loose? whooping? in paroxysms?
- Vomits after cough?
- Brings up sputum?   if so, foul smell?
● If swelling of face or body
- Passing urine as before (may be nephritis)?
- Colour of urine?
- Hair sparse, skin light and peeling?
- Getting pale, and gets out of breath?
● If fever
- For how long?
- What treatment given?
- Takes antimalarials?
- Any convulsions?
● If convulsion
- The *first* in his life?   if not, how often before?
- How long did the convulsion last?
- What was it like?
- Has he ever taken drugs for this?
- Did it occur with high fever?   anyone else in the family with a tendency to have seizures accompanying fever?
● If not sucking
- Was baby sucking before?
- Born or circumcised at home?
- Immature?
- Any spasms?

3

● If fast breathing
− Cough?
− How fed?
− Choked on food?
● If measles
− What day did fever start?
− What day did rash start?
− Is the child drinking?   or refusing?
− What are the stools like?

When finished

Ask 'Is there anything else you want to tell me?'

Simple physical examination

With a little training most people can become competent at clinical assessment by doing the following examinations.

1   Child's age, weight, weight assessment. If weighing scales are not available measure the arm circumference. Ideally height should also be taken.

2   Temperature, pulse (or apex beat rate in small infants), respiration.
● These are the neglected but **vital signs**.
● If recorded **on admission**, they can be used to assess progress.
● It takes **practice** to count children's pulses and infant's apex beats, but **it can be done**.

3   Appearance: what you learn by simply looking and touching gently.
● Behaviour: Happy? Peaceful? Miserable? Anxious? Distressed?   Unconscious or drowsy?
● General appearance: Looks ill? Well? Dehydrated? Listless?   Laboured breathing?   Pale?
● Nutritional state: Wasted?   Oedema?   Hair sparse?
● Skin: Rash? Cyanosis? Infection? Abscess? Peeling?

● Head:

Hair – normal?

Anterior fontanelle – bulging or sunken?

Eyes – sunken? staring? inflamed?

Nose – discharge? flaring?

● Chest: Respirations rapid? Indrawing? Abnormal shape?

● Abdomen: Distended? Tender? Swellings?

● Arms and legs: Swellings? Swelling of fingers?

● Back and buttocks: Spine straight? Abscess on buttocks?

4 Examinations which disturb child more: Leave to the end.

● Abdomen: Feel size of spleen and liver – mass? Bladder palpable?

● Eyes: Evert lower lid to assess anaemia – infected?

● Mouth: Evert lower lip – colour? Using a spatula, note teeth, gums, throat, palate. Koplik spots?

● Ears: Discharge, or inflamed tympanic membrane?

● Any other area that appears tender?

● See any recent vomit or stool if possible.

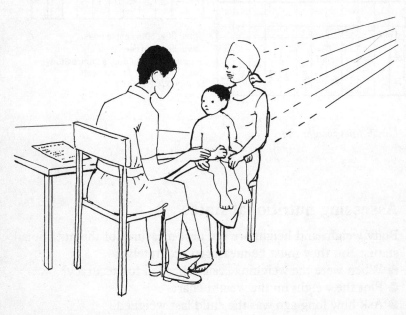

Examining a young child

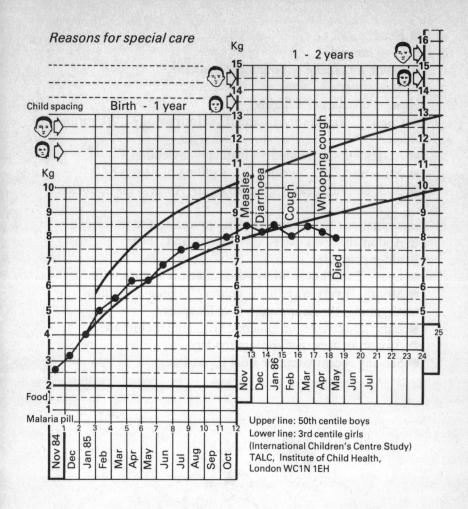

Reasons for special care

Child spacing

Birth - 1 year

1 - 2 years

Kg

Food
Malaria pill

Upper line: 50th centile boys
Lower line: 3rd centile girls
(International Children's Centre Study)
TALC, Institute of Child Health,
London WC1N 1EH

Under fives weight chart

Assessing nutritional status

Body weight and height are the best measures of the nutritional
status. But they must be measured accurately.

● When were the weighing scales checked for accuracy?
● Plot the weight on the weight chart.
● Ask how long ago was the child last weighed.
● Does the child possess his own weight card?

- Is the face swollen?   and the legs?
- Is the hair sparse or discoloured?
- Does the child see well at night?
- Is the mouth sore?

Measuring malnutrition by arm circumference

This is a useful indicator of malnutrition. The arm circumference also identifies severely malnourished children whose stunted condition makes their weight appear normal for their height. Its use is based on the fact that the mid-arm circumference increases by only about 1 cm between 1 year and 5 years of age. The same measurement then can be used throughout this period.

Table 1.1

Arm circumference	Indicates
Over 13.5 cm	Most children normal.
12.5 − 13.5 cm	Some children have mild malnutrition but no child with severe malnutrition.
Under 12.5 cm	Severe malnutrition. No child whose weight exceeded 80% weight-for-age in a test group had an arm circumference of more than 12.5 cm.

Circumference is *measured* by a fibre tape or a marked strip of X-ray film placed around the middle of the relaxed upper arm. The film strip can be coloured green, yellow and red to indicate the above 3 lengths.

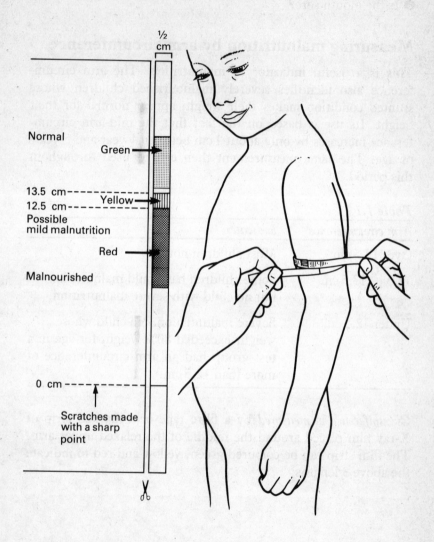

Normal

Green →

13.5 cm ---------
                    Yellow →
12.5 cm ---------
Possible
mild malnutrition

Red →

Malnourished

0 cm ---------
          ↑
Scratches made
with a sharp
point

Arm circumference

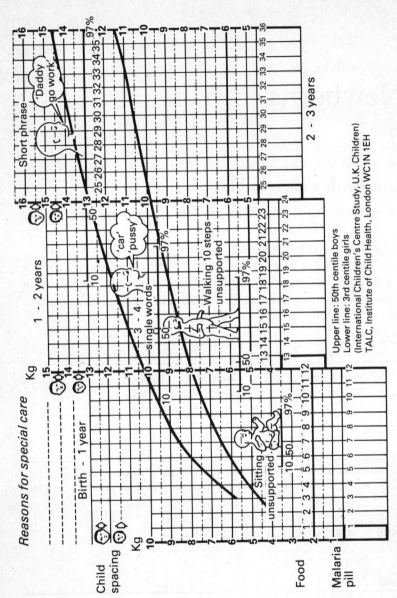

9

● CHAPTER 2

Newborns

Low birth weight babies

Babies weighing 2.5 kg (5½ lbs) or less at birth are described as low birth weight babies.

● About ⅓ are **pre-term**, born before 37–38 weeks gestation.
● ⅔ are **small for dates**, weighing less than they should for the gestation i.e. less than 10th centile weight due to failure of adequate growth in foetal life largely due to foetal malnutrition.

Table 2.1

Weeks gestation	*10th centile weight in g*[*]
36	2000
37	2200
38	2400
39	2600
40	2650

[*] If 100 babies of same gestation were put in order of weight, from low to high, the 10th centile is the weight of the baby 10th from the lowest weight.

Note   *Average* weights and lengths are:

Table 2.2

Weeks gestation	*Weight in g*	*Length cm*
28	1000	40
32	2000	44
36	3000	48

Main problems in the low birth weight babies

Table 2.3

Problem	Preterm	Small for dates
1 Respiratory	More common a few hours after birth – apnoeic attacks or respiratory distress.	Tendency to asphyxia at birth (due to oxygen lack in utero).
2 Heat regulation	Difficulty in maintaining temperature.	Some difficulty in maintaining normal temperature.
3 Feeding	Poor or absent sucking reflex resulting in: – starvation; – hypoglycaemia; – later – physiological jaundice.	Usually suck well. Sometimes aspirate feeds.
4 Infection	Very liable to infection.	Not such a great problem.
5 Hypo-glycaemia	Many develop if feeding insufficient.	Quite likely to develop.
6 Anaemia	Develops in smaller babies after 3–4 weeks	—

Routine special care of low birth weight babies

Labour ward staff
● Be prepared. Warn nursery staff too.
● Episiotomy to prevent intracranial damage.
● Ready with warmed towels.
● Ready for resuscitation.

11

To preserve body heat
● Act quickly! Remove wet delivery towels and replace with dry towel and blankets.
● Keep head covered.
● Hot water bottles if necessary.
● *Wipe* baby clean — don't *wash*.
● Check temperature (axillary) and chart.
— Aim to keep above 97°F (36°C).
— Check temperature hourly for first 12 hours, then 3–4 hourly, *and chart on graph*.
— If it goes below 97°F (36°C) warm up and check ¼ hourly until normal.
● Place in a warm nursery in a cot warmed with 2–3 well covered hot water bottles if close observation is required. All other low birth weight babies must go next to the mother, well wrapped up in a warm bed.

Note Incubators can be source of infection unless cleaning instructions are meticulously followed.

Deaths in infants weighing less than 1500 g can be reduced by a quarter or more if their body temperature is maintained above 36°C and care is taken to reduce heat loss to a minimum. Table 2.4 gives the room temperature necessary for maintaining body heat in small babies.

Table 2.4

Room temperature necessary to maintain body heat in small babies nursed, fully clothed and well wrapped in a cot in a draught-free room with moderate humidity.

Birth weight	Room temperature 29.5°C	26.5°C	24°C
1.0 kg	for 2 weeks ⟶	after 2 weeks ⟶	after 1 month
1.5 kg	for 2 days ⟶	after 2 days ⟶	after 2 weeks
2.0 kg	—	for 1 week ⟶	after 1 week
3.0 kg	—	for 1 day ⟶	after 1 day

Source Hey, E., *Br. J. Hosp. Med.* 1972

12

Have resuscitation equipment ready before delivery
- Suck out pharynx and also empty stomach to prevent regurgitation and aspiration. Mouth-to-mouth breathing (rate 20/min.) and external cardiac massage if necessary. (See pages 19–20.)
- When respiration established, check frequently for first few hours. Keep ½ hourly respiration chart.
- Do not give oxygen routinely unless there is apnoea or rapid breathing. Respiratory rate of more than 50 per minute after the second hour of birth should be regarded with suspicion and investigations considered.
- Position: best lying on side or prone with head to one side. *Turn* baby every 2–3 hours.
- Apnoea occurs in about a quarter of all pre-term babies. If severe and recurrent, treatment with theophylline 2 mg/kg every 8 hours orally should be considered.

To prevent bleeding
- Give Vitamin K_1 1mg I.M.

Feeding
- In the past feeding used to be started too late and was often insufficient. *Early* and *adequate* feeding with breast milk:
- reduces weight loss and helps growth;
- reduces incidence of hypoglycaemia and other metabolic abnormalities;
- reduces severity of physiological jaundice in prematures.
- Babies who can suck and swallow should breast feed and stay with their mothers. Their presence with her reduces anxiety and helps the milk flow. Those who cannot suck require tube feeding (diameter 3.5 F.G.) and later feeding by cup and spoon if able, but presence of sucking reflex should be looked for every day. Put to breast as soon as the reflex appears even though it may be weak and baby needs extra feeds.

What feeds to offer?
- Mother's milk as soon as possible after birth. Initial glucose feeds or water are not necessary even in hot climates.
- If not sucking, undiluted expressed breast milk (E.B.M.) Remember colostrum is normal and essential.

● If no E.B.M. available, consider milk from other mothers or other lactating women in the family. Artificial feeding is not needed and can be dangerous.

Times   How often?
● Start soon after birth, but within an hour or so.
● Feed 3 hourly − 8 feeds/24 hours.
● Or 2 hourly day and 3 hourly night − 11 feeds/24 hours depending on weight.

What amounts?
● If the baby can suckle well he should be able to obtain his daily requirements. Table 2.5 is intended for those who cannot suckle.

Table 2.5

Day	Expressed breast milk ml/kg/24 hours*
1	40
2	60
3	80
4	100
5	100
6	120
7	120
8	140
9	140
10	160
11	160
12	180
13	180
14	200

*No dilution is needed

Examples
● 2 kg baby 7 days old.
  Give 2 × 120 ml = 240 ml/24 hours.

  Fed 3 hourly $= \dfrac{240}{8}$

  $= 30$ ml/feed.

- 1.3 kg baby 3 days old.

  $1.3 \times 80 = 104$ ml/24 hours.

  Fed 11 feeds/day $= \dfrac{104}{11}$

  $\qquad\qquad\qquad = 10$ ml/feed.

To prevent infection
- Exercise special care.
- Wash hands before handling baby.
- Do not allow *anyone* with infection near baby.
- Each baby to have own thermometer and other items. Communal bath tubs and changing tables are common sources of infection.
- All ill babies should be nursed separately from the healthy ones.

To prevent anaemia
- Give ferrous sulphate orally for infants (30 mgm) and folic acid 0.5 mg/kg once a day from 2 weeks.

To prevent vitamin deficiency
- Give – Vitamin A   2500 i.u. ⎫
  - Vitamin D   400 i.u. ⎬ daily from the age of 2 weeks.
  - Vitamin C   25 mgm ⎭
- Check your preparation and work out your dose.

Low birth weight babies *need to feel secure* and it is good for the mothers to be with them all the time. Those in incubators or in a special care nursery are most likely to feel this insecurity. Such babies should come out as soon as fit and be given to their mothers to hold and cuddle even for short periods.

Low birth weight babies born at home

- If admitted to children's ward, nurse in a separate room for first 2 to 3 days to ensure that they do not bring in infection.
- **Cold** is a big problem and a *4 hourly temperature* chart essential for all. If initial temperature is subnormal, start $\frac{1}{2}$ hourly temperature chart until normal. The best way to warm up is to

let the mother hold the baby. The baby should be nursed in the same bed as the mother, both well covered with blankets.
- Give A.T.S. 350 units after test dose routinely. Antibiotics for 4–5 days as likelihood of infection in home delivery is very high.
- Feed as soon as possible after admission because if unable to suck must have been starving at home.

Note   All babies, however small or sick, should be weighed within 4 hours of birth or admission.

Asphyxia of the newborn

Most neonates breathe spontaneously, or after stimulation caused by the catheter when being suctioned. In a few cases the respiratory centre is not functioning well because of:
- shortage of oxygen during labour or delivery;
- physical injury to head during birth;
- respiratory depression due to drugs given to the mother in the few hours before birth, e.g. pethidine, morphine, anaesthetics or traditional remedies administered at home.

The condition of the baby is assessed by the **Apgar** Score at 1 minute and 5 minutes.

Table 2.6

Sign	0	1	2
Respirations	nil	slow – irregular	normal
Heart rate	nil	less than 100	more than 100
Colour	blue, pale	limbs blue	normal
Tone	limp	some flexion of limbs	active movement
Response to stimulus	nil	grimace or movement	cry

Score: Normal   8–10
        Moderate to mild asphyxia   3–7
        Severe asphyxia   below 3
A low score at 5 minutes is more serious than at 1 minute.

Equipment for neonatal resuscitation

● It is vital to **be ready**.
● It is also vital to keep the baby **warm** – so have warmed towels, hot water bottles or, if there is electricity, a 100 watt bulb light fitted so that it is 45–50 cm above the baby. An angle-poise lamp is most useful.

Even a rural clinic should have
● Slanted table.
● Towels and blanket.
● Mucus catheter.
● Piece of gauze (for mouth-to-mouth breathing).
● Chart for vital signs.
● If you give pethidine to mothers have naloxone available.
● 1 or 2 × 2 ml syringes.

And ideally
● Neonatal resuscitator.
● Infant airway size 0,00.
● Vitamin K injection.

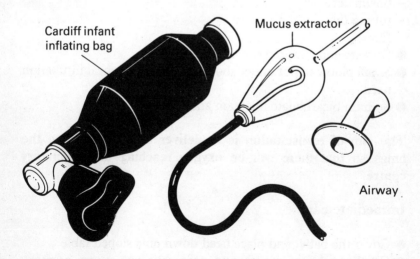

Cardiff infant inflating bag

Mucus extractor

Airway

Resuscitation equipment for a rural hospital

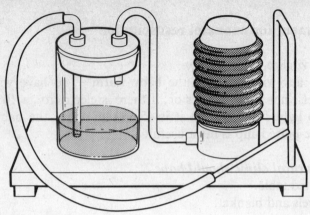

Foot suction pump

Hospitals should also have

● Mechanical suction e.g. Ambu.
● Suction catheters size 15 F.G.
● Laryngoscope with neonatal blade.
● Spare batteries.
● 3–4 neonatal endotracheal tubes – Warne's.
● Endotracheal connectors – Magill's. 0,00 including a T-shaped connector.
● Oxygen cylinder with
– flowmeter;
– tubing that fits connector;
– funnel.
● Scissors and strapping.
● Small pillow to put under shoulders if endotracheal intubation used.
● Sodium bicarbonate injection and 10 ml syringe.

The aim of resuscitation is to deliver air or oxygen to the lungs so that there will be oxygen reaching the respiratory centre.

Immediate care

● Cover the baby, and place head down on a sloped table.
● Gently suck out mouth and nose, but not strong *persistent* suction or else you suck out all the *air* too.

18

- Note Apgar.
- Most babies breathe satisfactorily.

If baby breathes or gasps but it is infrequent or inadequate
Aid respiration.
- If available, **oxygen by mask or funnel** (as long as there are some respirations), at the rate of 4 1/min.
- If available, use **neonatal resuscitator** – some models e.g. Blease Samson are designed for use *without* an infant airway, but with the head well extended. Others, e.g. Penlon are designed for use *with* airway. In most cases bag and mask resuscitation is suitable.
- If neither oxygen nor resuscitator available, do **mouth-to-mouth** respiration.
- Place gauze over baby's face.
- Extend head.
- Cover baby's nose and mouth with your mouth.
- Short puffs about 40/min. Use only the cheek muscles. Remember it is mouth-to-mouth *breathing* and not *blowing*.
- See chest expanding.
- Don't blow *too* hard as it can damage baby's lungs.
- If mother has recently received pethidine or morphine, give **naloxone** 60 mgm/kg I.V. or 200 mgm I.M. Give Vitamin K 0.5 mg.

Initial resuscitative measures like suction and administration of oxygen will initiate a gasp in 85% of cases.

If no respirations after 2–3 minutes or if initial gasps and then breathing stops
- Make sure the pharynx is clear of mucus or liquor.
- If resuscitator available, use. If you *see* chest expanding and *hear* air going into the lungs you are being effective. If there is improvement the heart rate will increase to over 100/min.
- If you have oxygen, attach to attachment on resuscitator.
- If no resuscitator available, carry out mouth-to-mouth breathing.

If still does not respond after 5 minutes
- Call for specialist help if there is another person available. Do

not stop the resuscitation to go looking for help if alone.
● Suction pharynx under direct vision using laryngoscope, if necessary.
● Such babies may need to have an endotracheal tube passed and strapped in position for prolonged aeration.

If no heart beat felt
● Do external cardiac massage. Two fingers mid sternum and press downwards gently 100–200 times a minute, while someone else continues to ensure air or oxygen to the lungs. Remember it is cardiac *massage* and not *squeeze*. Be gentle.

If baby still limp and not responding
● Give sodium bicarbonate 5–10 mEq by umbilical vein.

Follow up

● Keep warm and check that you are succeeding, by checking temperature every 15 minutes while resuscitation continues.
● If using resuscitator or endotracheal tube check both lungs for adequate air entry and heart rate. Slowing of heart rate indicates deterioration.
● Note time of:
– *1st* respiration;
– regular respirations.
● If mouth-to-mouth breathing was administered, start antibiotics.
● When breathing commences put baby head end up on the table or in the cot.

Most important Resuscitation *must be* continuous. Brain damage occurs if you walk away and leave the baby for 2–3 minutes. Do not go away until someone takes over from you.

How long should one continue resuscitation?

● If the heart is beating? As long as heart rate is over 100 continue as long as heart beat persists. If heart rate is persistently below 100 in spite of adequate resuscitation the outlook is poor – try for 20–30 minutes.

20

● If there is persistent cyanosis, slow heart rate and especially if the baby has been left for some minutes, the outlook is bad.

Other procedures

● Nikethamide and lobeline, drugs used in the past, are *not* advised — they can be dangerous.
● Slapping the baby's back and applying hot and cold water are *out*.

Remember   **Primary aim is to deliver oxygen to the brain.**

Lastly   after Caesarean section suck out the *stomach* as well as the pharynx, so that the baby will not regurgitate and aspirate stomach contents.

'Cerebral' babies

These are babies who show vague neurological signs and symptoms.

In first 48 hours

Clinically
● Hyperactive — or, if more severe, limp.
● Hypertonic.
● High pitched cry.
● Refusing to suck, or feeding with difficulty and vomiting.
● Unusual eye movements present occasionally.
● Twitching at times.

Occurs
After long — or precipitate labours — difficult or instrumental deliveries.

Treatment in first 48 hours
Rule out hypoglycaemia by doing Dextrostix test — and repeating it.

Table 2.7 Respiratory distress (after initial respirations established)

Characterised by	Possibly due to	More common in	Investigate	Treat
Sudden cessation of breathing. Gasping. Cyanosis.	Aspiration of mucus or stomach contents.	Low birth weight babies. Babies of diabetic mothers. Could be any baby.	—	Immediate suction. Lie baby on side. Antibiotics if aspiration pneumonia is suspected.
	Hypoglycaemia.	Small for dates babies. Low birth weight babies fed late and little.	Dextrostix. If less than 40 mgm measure blood sugar.	Treat as for hypoglycaemia.
	Intracranial haemorrhage.	Immature babies. After difficult or prolonged labour.	Examination of baby – 'cerebral'.	Gentle handling. Suction. Nasogastric feeding.
Respiratory rate rising – more than 60. Indrawing intercostals. Cyanosis, possibly grunting. Starting within 4 hours of birth.	Hyalin membrane disease.	Immature babies. After Caesarean section. Babies of diabetic mothers.	Examine baby. Possibly X-ray (usually few changes seen).	Feed by nasogastric tube. Hourly observations. Oxygen if and when cyanosed. If in doubt administer antibiotics. If severe insert umbilical catheter. I.V. 10% dextrose water 75 ml/kg/24 hours.

Characterised by	Possibly due to	More common in	Investigate	Treat
Starting 4 hours after birth.	**Pneumonia.**	Membranes ruptured more than 24 hours. Prolonged or instrumental labour. Infected at resuscitation.		Antibiotics. Suction if necessary. Turn from side to side 2–3 hourly.
	Congenital heart disease.	Any baby could have.	Apex beat usually rapid. Cardiac murmur present or absent. Liver usually enlarges. X-ray.	Treat cardiac failure if present, with digoxin and diuretic.
	Less common causes like congenital disease of the lung or diaphragmatic hernia.			Exclude other causes. Get specialist opinion.

Treat
- Sedation e.g. Diazepan 0.1 mgm/kg I.M. initially if twitching or restless then 0.5 mgm/kg 6−8 hourly and gradually decrease.

Or phenobarbitone 7.5 mgm 6−8 hourly.
- Nurse with head end up.
- Handle gently.
- Tube feed.

Symptoms occurring after first 48 hours

Consider meningitis and do lumbar puncture if in doubt.

Hypoglycaemia

Serious because it causes **brain damage.**

Occurs in first 2−4 days because of low reserve of glycogen in:
- small-for-dates babies;
- smaller of twins;
- babies of toxaemic mothers;
- some babies of diabetic mothers;
- and also in 'cold injury'.

Clinically
- Attacks of apnoea, pallor or cyanosis.
- Twitching and convulsions.
- Lethargy and poor muscle tone.

Prevent by early feeding (at 2 hours) and fuller feeding for low birth weight babies.

Watch out for by careful observation and by doing dextrostix 8−12 hours in likely babies.

Treat if blood sugar by dextrostix less than 30 mgm in full term and less than 20 mgm in small babies.
- If possible it is more reliable to do blood sugar in the laboratory − but do not delay treatment whilst awaiting results.

● **If no symptoms**
- Continue oral feeding and re-check dextrostix 6−8 hours later.
- If no increase in blood sugar give I.V. 10% glucose 75 ml/kg/24 hours.
● If hypoglycaemia **and symptoms**
- I.V. 50% glucose 1 ml/kg followed by:
- 10% glucose 75 ml/kg/24 hours and tail off slowly.
- Dextrostix 8 hourly.
- A few fail to respond and ACTH or cortisone may be ordered.
- Twitching or convulsions must *not* be allowed to continue.
- Give nasogastric feeds of expressed breast milk.

Procedures to be familiar with − Dextrostix
Note Always keep the cap of the dextrostix bottle on, and well on.

Dextrostix 1 minute test for glucose in whole blood
Before doing test, compare dextrostix with 'O' colour block on chart. Do not use if it does not match.

Note Protect strips from **light, moisture** and **excessive heat**.

● Store at 7°C and always under 30°C (86°F) − not in refrigerator.
● Keep bottle tightly capped.
● Remove only one strip for immediate use, leaving unused strips in bottle.
● Lay reagent strip on clean sheet of paper, not on table surface and not on absorbent towel.

Onset of symptoms

1 **Anoxia − from 1st day up to 3−4 days.**
2 **Hypoglycaemia − from 1st day up to 3−4 days.**
3 **Meningitis − from 3rd day and any day onwards.**
4 **Hypocalcaemia − not usually until 5th day.**
5 **Kernicterus − not usually until 5−6th day.**
6 **Tetanus − not usually until 6−7th day onwards.**

Table 2.8 Common causes of neonatal twitching or spasms

Cause	Diagnose by	Test	Treat
1 Anoxia	History of delivery – asphyxia. Presence of caput.	Dextrostix test normal.	Sedate. Nasogastric feeding. Head end up.
2 Hypoglycaemia	Low weight for dates.	Dextrostix. Blood sugar less than 30 mgm.	50% dextrose 1 ml/kg then 10% glucose 75 ml/kg/day I.V.
3 Meningitis	Leaking membranes? Long labour? Heart rate increased. Baby *looks* sick.	Lumbar puncture.	See treatment of *neonatal meningitis*.
4 Hypocalcaemia	Uncommon. Artificially fed baby. Occurs a few days after birth.	Spasm on tapping face in front of ear.	Calcium I.M. or orally.
5 Kernicterus	Severe jaundice. Haemolytic disease. G₆PD deficiency or A.B.O. incompatibility.	Bilirubin more than 20 mgm/100 ml.	Exchange transfusion. Sedate. Transfer if necessary.
6 Tetanus	Rarely before 6th day. Unable to suck. Risus sardonicus.	Examine baby.	Routine sedation and treatment.

Neonatal jaundice

Causes
- Physiological.
- Haemolysis.
- Infection.
- Certain drugs.
- Rare congenital causes.

Commonest cause
Physiological jaundice − occurs on 3−4th day (not before) and
clears by 6−8th day.
- Due to immaturity of the liver enzymes and therefore more
  severe in immature babies.
- Low birth weight babies with serum bilirubin levels above
  15−18 mgm% require exchange transfusion to avoid kernicterus.
- *Early* feeding (2−4 hours) with *sufficient* breast milk reduces
  the incidence and severity of physiological jaundice.
- Only treatment necessary − maintenance of an adequate milk
  intake, and adequate exposure to daylight.

**Jaundice in first 24 (even 36) hours is a neonatal emergency
and is due to haemolysis − breakdown of the red blood cells.**

Causes
- G_6PD deficiency commonest cause in many African countries.
- A.B.O. incompatibility − mother of blood group O is sen-
  sitised to baby who is either group A or B.
- Rh incompatibility which is rare in Africa.

Two newer methods found to reduce the bilirubin are now being
used, unless bilirubin is at critical level (18−20 mg/100 ml).
- **Phototherapy** − Baby is put under a fluorescent light or in
  diffuse daylight. Bilirubin is changed to another pigment,
  biliverdin. Baby should have eyes bandaged, extra fluids
  administered and hourly temperature checks to avoid over-
  heating.
- **Phenobarbitone** − 7 mgm orally 8 hourly reduces jaundice by

helping in the formation of the liver enzymes which deal with bilirubin. Remember to *stop* drug as soon as possible.

If the bilirubin is at or nearing 20 mgm%, this is the **danger level** and kernicterus may result. Clinically these babies have marked jaundice and 'cerebral' signs. The final result may be death or physical and mental handicap.

Dealing with neonatal jaundice

If mother seen antenatally. History of previous baby with severe neonatal jaundice
● Try to find cause from old chart.
● If no *facilities* for special tests and exchange transfusion – advise mother to deliver in special hospital or transfer baby and mother immediately after delivery.
● *If facilities available* – At delivery carry out the following investigations:
– Mother – blood group, Rh.
– Cord blood – bilirubin, haemoglobin, Coomb's test, blood group, Rhesus blood group and G_6PD level.
   1 If cord bilirubin at birth is over 5 mgm usually exchange transfusion is needed.
   2 If in doubt about ABO or Rh incompatibility use Gp O Rh.neg. blood – cross match with mother's serum.
   3 If cord bilirubin less than 5 mgm observe and check bilirubin 12 hourly.
   4 If jaundice increases treat with phototherapy and phenobarbitone. If rises to **danger level** do exchange transfusion.
   5 *After any exchange transfusion* check bilirubin 12 hourly until it is reducing safely.
   Retransfuse if at danger level.

If jaundice from birth to 24 (or 36) hours
● Take usual history and examine baby.
● Almost certainly due to haemolysis – due to ABO incompatibility, G_6PD deficiency or Rh incompatibility.
This is a neonatal emergency.
● *If no facilities available* – transfer baby and mother immediately after delivery.

28

- *If facilities available* − investigate in the following way.
- − Mother − blood group   Rh.
- − Baby − bilirubin, haemoglobin, Coombs test, blood group Rh, G_6PD test.

  1 If bilirubin at **danger level** i.e. approaching 20 mgm in full term or 18 mgm in low birth weight baby, do exchange transfusion.

  Also note (2) and (5) above.

  2 If bilirubin *not* at **danger level**, treat with phototherapy and phenobarbitone.

  Check 12 hourly and do exchange transfusion if bilirubin reaches **danger level**.

  Note (5) above.

In all
- Recheck Hgb/PCV every few days, may need simple blood transfusion later.

In G_6PD deficiency
- Explain to parents about the risk with certain drugs. Give 'certificate' to state baby has this condition.

In ABO incompatibility
- Explain to parents about chances of next baby having it. Need for antenatal investigations.

Jaundice starting after 36 hours

Causes
- **Physiological**
- **Infection**

Table 2.9

Associated with	Clinical signs	Action
Prolonged labour. Home deliveries. Difficult deliveries. Membranes ruptured for more than 24 hours. May be none of these.	Temperature up or low. Heart rate fast. Often discharging umbilicus or distended abdomen.	If possible culture swab from umbilicus and blood. Do lumbar puncture. **Antibiotics.** If bilirubin at danger level, exchange transfusion.

● G$_6$PD deficiency

Associated with	Clinical signs	Action
May be history of previous baby in family having jaundice. Maternal drugs.	Apart from jaundice baby looks well. *May* be associated *with* infection.	Question re drugs. Test for G$_6$PD deficiency. Check bilirubin every 12–24 hours. Stop any causative drug. Treat with phototherapy and phenobarbitone.

● **Certain drugs** e.g. chloramphenicol, Vitamin K, salicylates and sulfonamides can cause jaundice. Investigate and stop the drug.

● **Rarer causes**
  Congenital abnormalities of bile ducts
  – Jaundice starts later – usually in the second week.
  – It becomes gradually more marked.
  – Baby does not appear very affected in the first two weeks.
  – If near paediatric centre – transfer.
  Virus infections
  – These vary in severity.
  – Some are mild and though the jaundice persists for weeks, there is a gradual recovery.
  – Others are severe and associated with other clinical signs.

Note   Always do routine of history, examination and basic laboratory tests to **exclude *bacterial* infection** which you *can* treat.

Baby admitted after 48 hours – onset of jaundice not known

Cause
● Could be any of causes already mentioned or combination of them.

History
● Home delivery?
● Leaking membranes?

- Type of labour and delivery?
- Drugs – mother and baby?
- Any traditional remedies given to baby?

Clinically
- Weight L.B.W.
- Bulging fontanelle.
- Signs of infection.
- Signs of kernicterus.

Laboratory
- Minimal – bilirubin 12–24 hourly at first.
- Haemoglobin; PCV; leucocyte count; blood group; urine microscopy and culture if possible.
- **If infection** suspected – commence treatment with antibiotics.
- **If bilirubin** – 15 mgm or over, do tests for haemolytic disease and G_6PD if possible. **Watch for danger level** of bilirubin. If nearing it either transfer baby or treat.

In all
- Give phototherapy and possibly phenobarbitone.

If home delivery
- Antitetanus serum 350 units by subcutaneous injection.

Not passing urine

Possible causes
- Physiological.
- Baby *has* passed urine and no one saw.
- Poor fluid intake and resulting dehydration.
- Urethral obstruction (rare).
- Associated with meningomyelocoele – due to poor nerve control.
- In cardiac failure.

What to do
- Feel the napkin yourself – the baby may just have passed urine!

Common symptoms in the newborn period

Table 2.10 *Not sucking well or not sucking at all from birth*

Cause	Associated with	Treat by nasogastric feed and:
1 Immaturity	Maternal toxaemia, infections and many other causes.	Tube feed, until sucking reflex present.
2 'Cerebral' babies	Long or difficult deliveries. Instrumental delivery.	Elevate head end of cot. May need sedation.
3 Blocked nose	Sometimes after facial presentations.	Head end up. Nurse in supine position.
4 Cardiac failure	Severe congenital heart disease. Often associated with cyanosis and cardiac murmur – heart rate increased.	Treat with digoxin and diuretics.
5 'Cold' injury	Often after prolonged resuscitation.	Check temperature. Warm up; 4 hourly temperature chart.
6 Congenital defects Genetic defects	Hare lip. Severe C.N.S. defects.	May need tube feeding until operation.
7 Cretinism	Low temperature. Low cry.	If suspect – ask for specialist advice.

Table 2.11 Sucking well at first – then poor or no sucking

Cause	Associated with	Treat by nasogastric feed and:
1 Hypoglycaemia	Small for dates babies. Late or too little feeding.	Diagnose by dextrostix. Routine treatment for hypoglycaemia.
2 Nose blocked	Upper respiratory infection.	Saline nasal drops before feeds.
3 Neonatal tetanus	First sign. Usually born or circumcised at home.	Take history. Routine treatment of tetanus.
4 Cardiac failure	May start after some time. Heart rate over 160, increased respiratory rate and enlarging liver.	Chest X-rays and refer for specialist care. Digitalise and diuretic.
5 'Cold' injury	Can occur any time.	Warm up and follow well. Nurse the baby *near* mother; a good source of heat.
6 Any severe infection	e.g. pneumonia, meningitis, septicaemia.	Suspect since failure to suck is often the first sign. Investigate and treat.
7 Prolonged sedation	Hospitals. Someone orders sedation 6 hourly and no one remembers to stop it.	Always write sedation for a *certain number* of times.
8 Jaundice	Haemolytic disease of newborn.	Investigate cause and treat.
9 Anaemia	Often not obvious. Immature babies from 3 weeks onwards.	Measure haemoglobin and give either oral iron or imferon.

- Check on fluid intake − it may be poor.
- General check if baby:
− looks sick or in distress?
− apex beat normal?
− bladder palpable?
− meningomyelocoele?

You may have the answer if
- The baby looks sick, with or without cyanosis, with apex beat 150−200, increased respiratory rate and enlarged liver, consider cardiac failure.
- There is no abnormality and bladder not palpable. Plan a good fluid intake. Wait and see, the baby will pass urine.
- The bladder *is* palpable. Apply pressure gently and for some time in the suprapubic area. If the baby passes urine, recheck 6 hourly and inform doctor if the baby does not start passing urine spontaneously.
- After suprapubic pressure no urine is passed, ask those more experienced to see the baby. If they try and urine still not passed, it suggests **urethral obstruction**. Catheterisation with a suitably sized catheter and sterile precautions may be needed until the condition is investigated and treated.
  Note It is **rare**.

Not passing stool in neonate baby less than 48 hours old

Possible causes
- Normal delay.
- Imperforate anus.
- Congenital megacolon.
- *Some* babies with high obstruction.

What do you do?
- **Ask**
− If anyone else may have been present and seen meconium?
− Is there vomiting? − Is the baby feeding satisfactorily?
- **Look** at the baby
− Does he look ill − in distress?
− Is there abdominal distension − is it generalised or only in the upper abdomen? Is there obvious peristalsis seen?
− Can you pass a rectal thermometer?

Further steps
- If the anus is imperforate, send for the surgeon immediately.
- If vomiting, especially if there is also distension, suspect an obstruction. Ask for an X-ray (upright, abdominal film); carry out gastric aspiration and administer I.V. fluids whilst awaiting surgery.
- If normal anus, no vomiting, looks well, **Observe** and reassess.

Baby passes some meconium, then nil for 48 hours

Possible causes
- Normal baby.
- Congenital obstruction, e.g. atresia, bands.
- Other causes of obstruction, e.g. intussusception or meconium plug.

Note a baby with a congenital closure (atresia) of the gut may still pass meconium once or twice − and then stop passing anything per rectum.

Follow latter two steps above.

Loose frequent stools in neonate

When mother is a patient in your hospital or clinic

- Mother and baby are already known to you. You know about the baby's feeding − presumably breast feeding.
- For some reason (e.g. very ill mother) the baby may be having artificial milk feeds made up in the hospital.

What do you do?
- **Ask** a few important questions.
- − How long?   How many?   What are they like?
- − Is there vomiting?
- − What feed?   If powdered milk, how much?
- − Where does the water for making feeds come from?
- − How is the feed prepared?
- **Look** at the baby.

- Is he ill?   Is he dehydrated?   Is he hungry?
- Does he look underfed or overfed?
- Look at the stool — and ask to see the next, too.
- Ask for number of stools to be recorded on chart.

After all this, you have formed some opinion
- Baby looks well.
- Feeding sounds satisfactory.
- Stool slightly loose only — **Observe**. Discuss with mother.

- Baby does not look so well.
- Mother may be giving water herself — source doubtful.
- Stool may be abnormally loose, large or frequent.
- Discuss with mother.
- Start with oral rehydration. (See page 73)
- If facilities available, do rectal swab for pathogenic *E. coli*.
- Avoid cross infection to other babies.
- Baby is already dehydrated. As well as above start I.V. fluids (see under Diarrhoea page 75).

Diarrhoea in the newborn is extremely dangerous.

When baby comes from outside the hospital

The chances that the baby has had or is having a feeding bottle are higher. The likelihood of infection is higher.

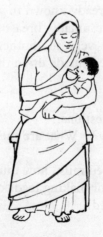

Feeding by cup

Follow routine as above.

- More need for **health education** to convince mothers of dangers of feeding bottle.
- If possible, try to establish breast feeding.
- If not possible, teach mother how to feed with cup and spoon, **or better still just the cup**.

Pallor or bleeding in neonates

Apparent
- Physiological e.g. vaginal bleeding.
- From the cord stump.
- Vomiting or bleeding per rectum (haemorrhagic disease).
- Bleeding from circumcision site.

} Presents as **bleeding**.

Hidden
- Through placenta into 2nd twin.
- Through placenta in ante partum haemorrhage.
- Cephalhaematoma or after prolonged vacuum application.
- Cerebral haemorrhage.
- Liver trauma (rare).
- As malaena.

} Presents as **pallor**.

Note
- Vaginal bleeding, usually 2nd−4th day, is physiological and is caused by maternal hormones. It will stop.
- Bleeding into the scalp after vacuum extraction occurs when the vacuum cup has been applied too long, or the pressure was increased too rapidly or was higher than advised.
- Cerebral haemorrhage, especially intraventricular haemorrhage, is more common in immature babies.
- Liver trauma, although rare, is more likely after breech delivery. The sudden pallor and shock usually occur a few *days* after delivery when the liver capsule finally ruptures. *Before* this happens a mass (the haematoma) may be palpable in the abdomen.

How to manage

Histo
- Twin? A.P.H.? Immature?
- Traumatic or instrumental delivery? Breech?
- Born at home and the cord not tied properly?
- Vomited blood or passed blood per rectum?

Examination
Note apex beat – temperature – respirations.
- In shock? Pallid? Immature? Weight?
- Looks cerebral? Head and scalp normal?
- Oozing from umbilicus or slipped cord ligature?
- Abdominal mass? Bleeding from circumcision site?
- Evidence of blood passed per rectum?

Laboratory investigations

Note

1 **Haemoglobin and packed cell volume levels** at this time are of no value as a measure of blood loss. (They will be in 24–48 hours and that might be too late.)
   General condition and heart rate indicate extent of blood loss.

2 **If blood loss severe** – baby critical.
   - Cross match group O Rh. negative blood with mother's serum as well as the baby's and give *stat*.
   - Blood taken at the same time may then be checked for haemoglobin/packed cell volume and grouping.
   - Baby will need more than usual 5 ml/kg and repeated small transfusions of packed cells may be needed.

3 **If blood loss not severe** and baby not critical.
   - Collect blood for grouping and cross matching and have blood ready.
   - Haemoglobin and packed cell volume estimations may be done to serve as baseline.

- Assess progress by checking heart rate every 15−30 minutes.

Treatment

In all
Indication for giving blood depends on the following factors.
- Amount of blood loss − when it can be seen.
- General condition of baby − especially a rising heart rate. Check apex rate every 10−15 minutes. If rising 140 → 160 → 180 (and baby not crying) it suggests continuing blood loss.

- If baby critical, save time, and the baby, by starting an I.V. infusion with dextrose water while waiting for the blood.
- If critical may be too weak to suck and need nasogastric feeding until improved.
- Keep the baby warm.

Bleeding from the umbilical stump
- Clamp and re-tie.
- If happened in your own hospital or clinic, reassess your method. Change to clamps or the new rubber band method?

Haemorrhagic disease of newborn
- Transfuse if indicated.
- Even if not critical, have blood ready − continue to check apex beat rate; at any time there may be another bleed.
- Vitamin K 1 mgm I.M. Repeat in 4−6 hours.

Bleeding circumcision
- Stop bleeding with mosquito forceps (or pressure).
- Suture.
- If circumcised at home, give penicillin intramuscularly for 3 days and A.T.S. 350 units subcutaneously.

Baby not moving an arm

Possible causes
- From **birth**
- Fracture of clavicle.

- Fracture of humerus.
- Brachial plexus (Erb's) palsy.
● **Later**
- Osteomyelitis.
- Septic arthritis.
- Sickle cell disease (in older infants).

Ask
● Difficult delivery, especially with the shoulders if vertex or with the arms if breech?
● Long labour with many vaginal examinations? Infected?
● Leaking membranes?

Examination
● Temperature? Pulse? Respiration and general appearance?
● Check for arm movements by doing Moro's reflex.
● Palpate clavicles by raising shoulders with your left hand, letting the head fall back, exposing the **clavicles**.
● Palpate upper arms for tender area of fracture of **humerus**.
- If the arm is limp with little or no pain on movement and the elbow is extended − this suggests **Erb's palsy**.
- If there is an area of tenderness and swelling − area feels warm and baby has a raised temperature − consider **osteomyelitis**.

Treatment
Fracture clavicle   Tell parents. It will not cause harm. Always lift the baby carefully, with hand supporting *back*. There will be a 'lump' there in a week. It is a sign of healing. It will go in 6−8 weeks.

Fracture humerus   Some leave alone. Others prefer to put a small soft pad in the axilla and strap affected arm to the body. It heals well.

Erb's palsy
● When in cot. Fix tape around wrist and pin to sheet as shown. This prevents deformities.
● Exercises. Hold baby's hand gently, place it on baby's abdomen, pass up over trunk to face, head, top of head, and then outwards through a full circle.
  Encourage mothers to do 10 times morning and evening.
● Most children recover fully. Reassure parents.

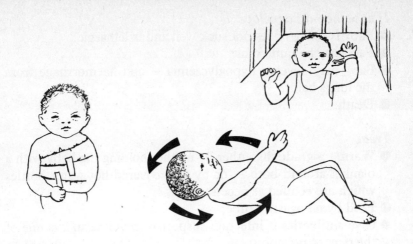

Fracture of the humerus   *Erb's palsy*

If infection is suspected (osteomyelitis or arthritis)
- X-ray area — but usually no changes for 7–10 days.
- Give antibiotics — usually penicillin *for 20–30 days*.
- Re-X-ray in 7–10 days.

Newborn hazards

Cold injury — hypothermia

This *can* and *does* happen in tropical countries, especially in:
- low birth weight babies;
- babies requiring resuscitation;
- babies with infections.

Prevent
- Do not allow baby to *become* cold after birth. Keep warm by drying and wrapping up immediately — and covering the head. The head is a relatively *large* area and much body heat can be lost from it.
- At night, especially in the cold of the wet season, wrap up well. Remember — mother is a wonderful source of warmth. Always keep the baby with the mother.
- Do not expose by bathing soon after birth.
- Use low reading thermometers to spot early hypothermia.

41

If hypothermia develops
- Baby is cold − does not suck well and is lethargic.
- Face may be quite pink.
- Baby may develop hypoglycaemia − and haemorrhage from the lungs before −
- Death.

Treat
- **Warm up gradually** either by mother holding the baby with a blanket around both − or by well covered hot water bottles **which are refilled** as necessary.
- Feed by nasogastric tube.
- Give antibiotics if infection suspected (hypothermia is one of the *signs* of infection).

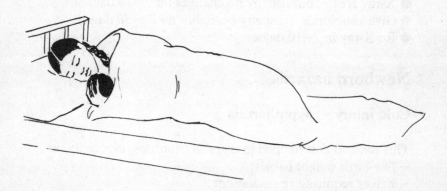

The best way

Notes on infection in the newborn

After delivery in maternity clinics and hospitals

Infection is usually not common because
- trained staff assist at delivery and
- mother and baby remain as a unit together so

- there is little cross infection, **but every now and then it happens**.
- It's unexpected — no one thinks of it, it's often not diagnosed until **it's very late or too late. Why?**

- The **awareness** of the **possibility of infection** has dropped and **awareness** of the **early signs** of infection is forgotten.

- The **possibility** of infection will be reduced if there is a **constant piped water supply**. This is possible in every rural clinic. Yet there are still many rural clinics without a constant water supply.
- Health workers have to *do* something to get this. It will not come without making others aware of the need.
- The clinic is also the place to teach **hygiene** to the mothers. They stay at the clinic a few days and have the time and the interest.
- **Serious infection** will be diagnosed if you are **aware of the early signs.**
- Main characteristics — vagueness of signs — at first:
- baby not sucking so well;
- looks paler than before;
- feels colder and temperature is low;
- *or* feels warmer and temperature is up a little;
- an occasional vomit;
- irritability — maybe;
- or lethargy;
- loose stools.
- If you examine the baby you may find:
- a full fontanelle;
- pustules, or discharging eyes, nose, or umbilicus;
- discharging ear;
- or *none* of these.
- You *will* find fast heart rate. This is one of the earliest signs.
- If you examine the urine — albumen? pus cells?

Later infection

Localised and obvious
- Abscesses, ophthalmia.

- Pneumonia with fast breathing, indrawing of intercostals and flaring nose.
- Meningitis with bulging anterior fontanelle.
- Gastroenteritis.

Generalised

- Tetanus − with spasms, inability to suck and risus.
- Septicaemia − with jaundice, distended abdomen, and going on to shock.

Think of sepsis in early rupture of membranes, prolonged labour with many vaginal examinations, especially if the birth was at home.

Treatment

1   Treat early − because the baby's resistance is low and infections spread fast in neonates, so treat at the **early signs**.

2   If facilities permit, investigate:
    - if pus present, take specimen for culture;
    - if in doubt about meningitis, do early **lumbar puncture**.

3   If no facilities − treat without delay.
    - **Infection diagnosed** − type unknown.

    It may be gram positive or gram negative organisms − give antibiotics which will cover both.
    - The most peripheral clinic will have penicillin and streptomycin. Penicillin 150 000 units daily or 6 hourly depending on severity, I.M. Streptomycin 100 mgm daily I.M. (half dose in low birth weight).
    - Gentamycin is a preferable alternative to streptomycin.
      Dose 3 mg/kg every 12 hours.
      Do not exceed this dose. Give for 4−5 days.
    - Ampicillin and cloxacillin combination may be kept for the *very* sick. It is expensive. If given to every baby there will soon be drug resistance.
      Dose Ampiclox (ampicillin 250 mg; cloxacillin 250 mg) 62.5 mgm 6−8 hourly I.M.

● **If diagnosed** as meningitis, septicaemia, peritonitis or any other severe infection.
– Give Ampiclox or gentamycin I.V. for some days.
● **If diarrhoea** commence oral rehydration. Check if the baby is entirely breast fed.
– In bottle fed babies consider neomycin 25 mgm/kg/day. Divide and give 12 hourly orally for 4–5 days.
● **If tetanus – see section on this.**
● **If localised swelling and tenderness of a limb are present, the most likely diagnosis is osteomyelitis** (but rule out fracture). Swelling and tenderness of shoulder, hip or knee suggests **septic arthritis** and often osteomyelitis also.
– Give penicillin in larger doses for 21 days continuing *even* after the swelling and tenderness go.
Otherwise it may recur.
● **If pus**, or suspected pus, do not delay incision. Always send pus swab for culture.

Neonates with infection admitted after home delivery

The incidence of infection here may be high – it averages 70% of neonatal admissions in some hospitals. Mortality is high – often up to 15%. These babies are usually very ill, and there is no question of 'early signs'.

Points to remember
● Jaundice and distended abdomen often indicate infection although both have other causes.
● Tetanus may be present *as well as* another obvious infection.
● Treat as already suggested, giving those antibiotics intravenously that can be given by that route every 6 hours as a bolus through a drip.
● If the I.V. needle goes into the tissues, **do not miss a dose of antibiotic**, give it I.M. Arrange to have I.V. restarted.
● Calculate fluid requirements and watch for over hydration.
● If infection occurred in hospital deliveries make a thorough investigation of the cause. Avoid communal bath tubs, changing tables, soaps, towels. Always keep the baby with the mother; not in a separate nursery. Insist on breast

feeding. The milk kitchen is a common cause of gastro-enteritis in the newborn.

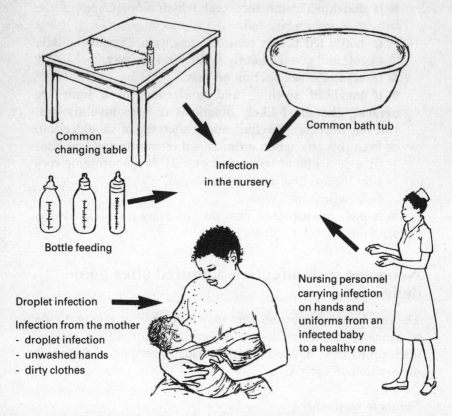

Common changing table

Common bath tub

Infection in the nursery

Bottle feeding

Droplet infection

Infection from the mother
- droplet infection
- unwashed hands
- dirty clothes

Nursing personnel carrying infection on hands and uniforms from an infected baby to a healthy one

Avoid all these. They can cause infection in the nursery

Hazards to neonates on I.V. fluids

It *is* a hazard for a neonate to be at the receiving end of an I.V. infusion of normal saline or dextrose saline.

Full strength Darrows solution is even more hazardous, but not so commonly used, probably as it is in shorter supply.

Why?

● Neonates cannot excrete sodium chloride (saline) and potassium (as in Darrows) very efficiently.

- If sodium, chloride and potassium are being poured into the veins through an I.V. drip, and only very little is excreted through the kidneys, then the blood levels of sodium, chloride and potassium rise to danger levels **very quickly**.
- High blood levels of sodium cause convulsions and later death: if the baby lives there may be permanent brain damage.
- High blood levels of potassium affect the heart and can also cause death.

Treatment of dehydrated neonates

In the clinic or peripheral hospital situation it is best to have some general rules.

1 Start an I.V. drip 5% dextrose in N/5 saline, take a history and examine the baby. Decide on probable cause of dehydration.

2 Calculate fluid requirement:
Wt in kg × 20 = ml given fast (e.g. 20 mins.)
then 25 ml/hour for 24 hours.
e.g. 3 kg baby − 60 ml fast
                            600 ml in 24 hours.

3 ● If dehydration is due mainly to *diarrhoea*, the baby needs *some* potassium, sodium and chloride to replace what is lost in the stool.
   ● Oral rehydration can be carried out using equal volumes of water alternately with sugar/salt solution.
   ● If severely dehydrated start with Hartman's solution intravenously. Re-assess after 4 hours. See plan C on page 75..
   ● **Second 24 hours** The baby should be well hydrated and breast feeding. If not, continue oral rehydration and breast feeding.

4 ● If dehydration only due to **insufficient fluid intake** e.g. motherless baby, calculate requirements as above.
   ● If mild − try fluids orally by cup or cup and spoon.
   ● If moderate and baby too weak to drink, give nasogastric drip and observe hourly.
   ● If severe give Hartman's solution intravenously *and* milk by nasogastric route.

Hazards of care by untrained traditional birth attendant

'Hazards' because babies delivered by untrained traditional midwife would not have had the best care antenatally or at delivery.

Table 2.12

Because	Result
At delivery	
● Primigravidae tend to be very young.	Disproportion – obstructed labour – **birth trauma** and **asphyxia**.
● Local midwives do not understand sepsis.	Mother **infected** when vaginal examination done – sometimes baby also infected.
● Mother may have something inserted in vagina, often infected with tetanus (e.g. sticks).	Baby gets **tetanus**.
● Mother may be given native oxytocic medicine.	Uterus in tonic contraction – **foetal asphyxia**.
● Mother has malaria.	**Premature** delivery and **low birth weight**.
● Mother has infection e.g. gonorrhoea.	Baby develops **ophthalmia neonatorum**.
● Mother has anaemia.	Baby has poor iron stores and likely to develop anaemia in infancy.
Baby	
● Applications to cord.	**Tetanus, generalised infection.**
● Applications to eyes.	**Conjunctivitis.**
● Circumcision in male.	**Bleeding, infection, tetanus.**
● Circumcision in female.	As above and narrowing of introitus.
● Hand feeding.	Baby **aspirates** – baby infected.
● Put on mother's back before can hold head up.	**Regurgitates** and **aspirates**.
● Native enemas.	Sometimes cause death due to **water intoxication** or **dehydration**.
Prevention	
● Proper antenatal care at maternity clinics.	Should *reduce*:
● Hospital care for special patients.	– birth trauma;
● Basic training for traditional birth attendants.	– many cases of asphyxia; – infection; – premature delivery;
● Proper newborn care and health education.	– hazards to baby.

Newborn care

Well described in 'Care of the Newborn in Developing Countries' by G.J. Ebrahim. Available from Teaching Aids at Low Cost (TALC) and Macmillan Press Ltd. Small, clear and good for teaching.

Health education during the time a mother is admitted for delivery

● Before you teach *anything*, find out customs in your area.
● Mention good ones also, so as not to be always criticising e.g. breast feeding, love of babies, babies with the mother are happier people.

Preventing hazards

● **Applications to cord**. Why is it done in a specific area? Probably a reason, e.g. earth applied to make baby one with ancestors who are in the earth. Give *alternative* to apply. Do not say 'Never apply anything'. Some use mercurochrome or triple dye for example — it can be *seen*.

● **Application to eyes**. Some put breast milk in eyes. Find out why. Could ask patients if they have had milk in their eyes?

● **Circumcision in the male**. Very traditional. If you can train nurse or medical assistant, circumcision will be done in a safe and sterile way. Giving tetanus toxoid to mother in pregnancy will prevent the occurrence of tetanus.

● **Circumcision in female**. Sometimes done in neonatal period. Sometimes at puberty. Suggest you really fight this. It is done often so as to remove the clitoris and it is said by some people that men think women will be more faithful to their husbands if this is done, as they do not get enjoyment from intercourse. The following complications can occur:
− death from blood loss;
− infection including tetanus;
− scarring and difficult delivery later.
Explain all this to the women and as they become educated the custom will, it is hoped, die out.

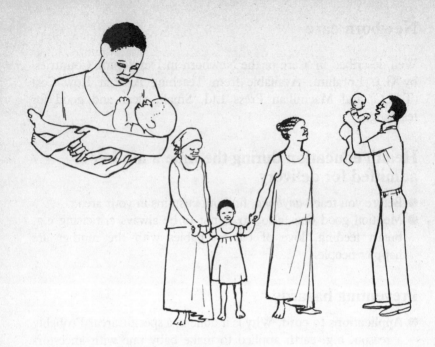

Good traditions (above). Bad traditions (below)

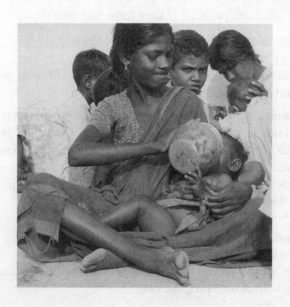

- **Hand feeding**. Done in certain areas. Baby held almost up-side down between mother's legs and fluid poured into mouth. Result, asphyxiation, pneumonia and often death.
- **Tied on to mother's back** before able to hold head up. Explain to the mothers and grandmothers – they often understand when told.
- **Native enemas** from one week of age. A hard custom to stop. Babies die of water intoxication, or are admitted with grossly distended abdomens – explain the dangers.
- There will be others – some good – some not so good.

Babies admitted from home

- If admitted to the children's ward, keep cot away from window *or* shut the window to avoid draught and cooling.
- **Cold** is a big problem and **4 hourly temperature** chart essential for all. If initial temperature subnormal, start $\frac{1}{2}$ hourly temperature chart until normal.
- If born *at home* give:
- A.T.S. 350 units;
- antibiotics for 4–5 days as likelihood of infection in home delivery is very high.
- Feed as soon as possible after admission because if unable to suck, must have been starving at home.

Note All babies, however small or sick, should be weighed within 4 hours of birth or admission.

Some congenital malformations requiring emergency treatment

Table 2.13

Clinically	Possible diagnosis	To do
Chin very receding. Choking spells and attacks of cyanosis.	Micrognathia.	Nurse in semi-prone position so that the tongue does not block pharynx.
Unable to suck or regurgitating through nose.	Hare lip. Cleft palate.	Tube feed or feed with cup and spoon. Operation – hare lip 2–3 months.

51

Table 2.13 (contd.)

Clinically	Possible diagnosis	To do
Vomiting – persistent in first few days. Not more than one or two stools. Possibly abdominal distension.	Intestinal obstruction? Duodenal or jejunal atresia.	1 Insert nasogastric tube and suction hourly. 2 I.V. fluids. 3 See surgeon.
Attacks of cyanosis after feeding. Mucus + + from mouth.	Tracheo – oesophageal fistula.	Refer to nearest large centre for corrective surgery. Tube feed if possible.
Abdominal organs 'herniated' into umbilicus.	Exomphalos.	1 Nasogastric tube and suction $\frac{1}{2}$ hourly. 2 See surgeon immediately. 3 Sterile dressing.
Not passing meconium or stool.	Obstructed? Imperforate anus?	Refer for surgery.
Signs of cardiac failure. Enlarging liver, tachycardia, possibly oedema, cyanosis.	Congenital heart disease.	Refer to specialist. Digitalise and give diuretic.

Treatment required – but not emergency
Table 2.14

Clinically	Possible diagnosis	To do
Extra digits.		Tie small ones off at base. If bony, see surgeon.
Abnormality of lumbar spine. Spina bifida.	Meningomyelocoele. Possibly hydrocephalus.	Cover with sterile dressing. Refer to surgeon.
Urethral opening in unusual place.	Hypospadias.	Do not circumcise. Skin required *for operation later*.

52

Clinically	Possible diagnosis	To do
Unable to fully abduct hips.	Congenital dislocation of hip.	Send to orthopaedic surgeon.
Foot turns in and points downwards.	Talipes or 'Club foot'.	1 See if *mobile* by touching sole of foot. If it is, show mother how to place foot in normal position. Do 10 times a.m., noon, p.m. 2 If will not go into good position, **see doctor as soon as possible**. Should have treatment **in first** 4–5 days. 3 If seen later **still send immediately to doctor**. He may refer child to orthopaedic surgeon and prevent crippling for life.
Blindness.	1 Eye tumour. 2 Congenital cataract.	See eye specialist immediately.

Neonatal emergencies in first 48 hours

You *can* diagnose neonatal emergencies and save many lives.
To do this you must:
● be familiar with the possibilities;
● take certain basic steps to make the diagnosis;
– take detailed history of pregnancy and labour,
– observe the baby undressed and do full physical examination,
– have certain diagnostic aids to hand,
● know where to refer the babies if they present with emergencies in rural clinics;
● not waste time.
You can *prevent* many neonatal emergencies. To do this you must:
● be familiar with the *kind of baby* who may get into trouble;
● carry out certain routines that will *prevent* trouble;
● recognise the *earliest signs* of trouble.

53

Table 2.15 *Neonatal emergencies in first 48 hours (excluding birth asphyxia)*

At initial examination after birth

Clinically	Cause	Occurs in	Steps to be carried out
Pallor.	Blood loss before or during delivery.	● Caesarean section. ● 2nd twin. ● Antepartum haemorrhage.	Blood transfusion with group O Rh negative blood up to 10–12 ml/kg.
Micrognathia.	Congenital abnormality.		Nurse in prone position to keep airway clear.
Exomphalos.	Congenital abnormality.		● Cover with dressing. ● Aspirate stomach. ● Transfer to hospital. Requires operation immediately.

During follow up observations

Clinically	Cause	Occurs in	Steps to be carried out
Bleeding from the cord.	A slipped ligature.		Clamp and re-tie. Transfuse if necessary.
Hypothermia: ● cold to touch; ● temperature below 97°F (36°C).	Delay in wrapping or too few coverings.	● Prematures. ● Those requiring resuscitation.	● Prevent. ● Hot water bottle. ● Cover head. ● Best when mother holds close to her body.
Ophthalmia Neonatorum – oedema and discharge from the eyes.	Gonococcal usually.	Infected mothers.	Intensive course of penicillin eye drops (5 000 units/ml) and I.M. penicillin.

Respiratory symptoms

Clinically	Cause	Occurs in	Steps to be carried out
Sudden cyanosis.	May be aspiration of mucus.	More common in immature.	Aspirate. Lie on side on flat surface.
Respiratory distress syndrome. Respiration more than 60. Indrawing intercostals. Grunting – Cyanosis within 4 hours of birth.	Hyaline membrane.	More common in 'small for dates' babies.	Keep warm. Feed by nasogastric tube. Oxygen if available – and if cyanosis. Antibiotics if question of infection.
Rapid respiration. Cyanosis occurring later than 4 hours.	May be pneumonia.	Membranes ruptured more than 24 hours. Prolonged labour. Infected at resuscitation.	Nurse prone. Keep clear airway. Turn from side to side. Antibiotics – penicillin and streptomycin, or gentamycin, or ampicillin and cloxacillin.

Table 2.15 (*contd.*)

Apparently central nervous system symptoms

Clinically	Cause	Occurs in	Steps to be carried out
Attacks of cyanosis, pallor, twitching. Generalised convulsions. Apnoea attacks.	● Cerebral hypoxia (in utero) or trauma or haemorrhage. ● Hypoglycaemia. Blood glucose below 20 mgm.	Prolonged or obstructed labour. Forceps delivery. Pre-term immature babies. 'Small for dates' babies. Toxaemia of pregnancy in mothers. Smaller of twins. Babies of diabetic mothers.	*Differentiate* by: ● history; ● Dextrostix test; ● examination. *Treat* If 'cerebral' sedate. If hypoglycaemic: − moderate − 10% glucose intragastric; − if below 20 mgm − I.V. glucose 50% 1 ml/kg then drip 10% 75 ml/kg/day. ● Breast feeding to commence as soon as possible.

Gastro-intestinal symptoms

Clinically	Cause	Occurs in	Steps to be carried out
Vomiting: ● persistent; ● large amount.	Obstruction: ● high – little distension; ● low – marked distension.	More common with polyhydramnios.	Keep warm. Aspirate stomach $\frac{1}{2}$ hourly. Arrange X-ray and surgery. Transport if necessary.
Distension.			
Stool – none or 1 or 2.			
Not sucking.	Immaturity. 'Cerebral'. Cardiac failure. (In congenital heart.) Choanal atresia. (Congenital block between nose and mouth.)	Pre-term. Difficult delivery.	Nasogastric feeding. Nasogastric feeding. Check apex beat rate and liver size. Treat with digoxin. Confirm diagnosis by inserting nasogastric tube. Keep airway in mouth.

57

Table 2.15 *(contd.)*

Jaundice first 24 (even 48) hours

Clinically	Cause	Occurs in	Steps to be carried out
Jaundice and pallor. Liver and spleen felt.	● G₆PD deficiency. ● A.B.O. incompatibility. ● Rh. incompatibility.	● Congenital deficiency. ● Sensitised mothers. ● Sensitised mothers.	If not in hospital transport *stat.* to a centre that can deal with the problem. ● Needs tests and exchange transfusion? ● Phototherapy for less severe.

Looking seriously ill but nothing specific

Clinically	Cause	Occurs in	Steps to be carried out
Not sucking well.	Infection.	Membranes ruptured a long time.	● In well-equipped hospitals culture – blood.
May be vomiting. Apex beat 160+. Temperature up or down. Colour may be pale.		Long labour. Interference. Mouth-to-mouth resuscitation.	● Lumbar puncture. ● Treat *stat.* Gentamicin or ampicillin and cloxacillin.

● CHAPTER 3

Tetanus

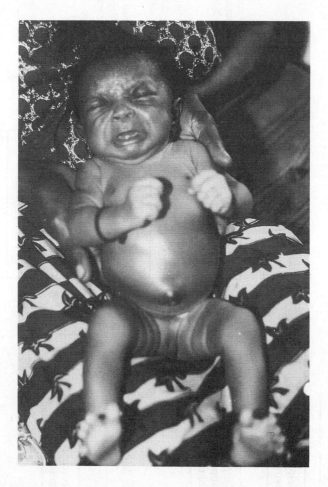

Neonatal tetanus

TETANUS – What we are aiming to do

Kill the organism.
Cl. tetanus.
— Penicillin first choice or tetracycline 1–6 days.

Help neutralise the toxin which causes spasms.
— Antitetanus serum 5000 units. Human tetanus immune globulin if available.

Keep the baby alive by supporting vital functions. Takes 3–4 weeks.

BREATHING
— Prevent spasms, but don't kill with oversedation – Give small repeated doses at regular 3 hourly intervals rather than few large doses.

GENERAL CARE
— Handle baby with care for washing and turning about ½ hour *after* sedation not when level of sedation light.

FEEDING
— Expressed breast milk by nasogastric tube – check progress by weight chart. Expect sucking reflex to return end of 3rd weeks.

IMMUNISE BABY
— 1st D.P.T. at 6–8 weeks.

Prevent it happening again.

IMMUNISE MOTHERS ANTENATALLY
— Tetanus toxoid injection at 32 and 36 weeks of pregnancy.

TEACH TRADITIONAL MIDWIVES
— Contact them in friendly way and help them.

Neonatal tetanus

Tell parents before admission that tetanus takes 3 or 4 weeks to get better otherwise they expect recovery in a few days and want to take the baby home when there is no rapid improvement.

History

- Antenatal care – Yes? No?
- If yes – where?
- Date of delivery. Where?
- If at home – name of midwife?
- Cord cut with . . . . ?
- Applications to the cord were . . . . ?
- Date of first symptom and type.
- Circumcised? What day?
- From these facts you can work out the incubation period, and if it is less than 5 days the prognosis is extremely serious.

Treatment

- **Sedate** immediately – paraldehyde 0.2 ml/kg intramuscularly.
- **20 minutes later**
- Insert a nasogastric tube and secure well.
- Give antitetanus serum 5 000 units intramuscularly. Alternatively antitetanus immunoglobulin 250 units intramuscularly has less risk of reaction, but is expensive and hard to obtain.
- Give crystalline penicillin 125 000 units (75 mg) intramuscularly and continue daily for 5–7 days or 2–4 times daily.

Sedation
- Dose depends on weight and severity of condition.
- Chlorpromazine 3–6 mg 6 hourly e.g. 6 am–12 noon–6 pm–12 mn through nasogastric tube.
- Diazepam 0.5 mg 6 hourly e.g. 9 am–3 pm–9 pm–3 am through nasogastric tube.
- Double dose may be required in the first 2–3 days.

Spasm chart
By checking the number and the severity of the spasms and the tone in the limbs once or twice a day either increase or decrease the sedation − but do not casually miss out doses. It is usually possible to stop one sedative drug in the third week and the other a little later.

Feeding
- Give expressed breast milk (EBM) if at all possible. Infants with tetanus can usually only tolerate small amounts the first day or two − about 75 ml/kg/day. Increase gradually over the next few days until the infant is given 150 ml/kg/day.
- Feed *slowly* − taking 20 minutes − as a rapid intragastric feed will cause regurgitation, aspiration and possible collapse and death. If the milk is cold, warm it slightly − cold milk passing down the tube causes spasms.

Weigh twice a week and chart.

Temperature
These are *neonates* and tend to get *cold*. So 4 hourly temperature check and act accordingly.

Turn from side to side as the mother will not think of doing this. If you do not the infant is likely to develop pneumonia.

Umbilical stump
- Clean very well on admission, and daily with soap and water. It will dry quicker if mercurochrome in spirit (or some similar preparation) is applied.
- It is better left **uncovered**.

Resuscitation
- Be prepared with:
- suction apparatus by cotside;
- neonatal resuscitator;
- endotracheal tube and laryngoscope (if you have them).

If collapse occurs
- Resuscitate first − and then try to find out the cause.

- If it happened during spasms it suggests *under* sedation.
- If it occured when the infant was very quiet — this suggests *over* sedation. Change medication accordingly.

Note   After 10–14 days babies will need less sedation.

Experience has shown that infants do better *near* the nurses' station where they can be observed night and day, **not** far away in a distant room.
It is **touch** that causes spasms — far more than noise or light.

Educate the mother about prevention
- For *this* baby — explain that having tetanus does not prevent it happening again. Give the first triple vaccine or tetanus toxoid before leaving hospital. Arrange 2 further injections at monthly intervals.
- For her *next* child — tell her of the value of 2 injections of tetanus toxoid during the antenatal period.

Children with tetanus

Clinical picture

- A recent wound, abrasion or scratch is not always seen.
- A recently pierced ear may be a point of entry of the infection.
- In our experience 20% of children had discharging ears.
- If there is trismus — check that a dental abscess is not the cause.
- If a painful stiff neck is present — differentiate from meningitis in which there is no trismus but the C.S.F. is abnormal.

Management

This is basically the same as for neonates.

Initial heavy sedation — if possible with paraldehyde
- 20–30 minutes later, insert nasogastric tube and secure well.
- If there is a wound clean well. Check for foreign body.
- Examine ears.
- Give initial dose of penicillin G and continue with procaine

penicillin daily intramuscularly 1 ml for 5—7 days.
- Give antitetanus serum — opinions differ as to the optimum dose.

Suggest at 1 year — 10 000 units;
                 5 years — 25 000 units;
             10 years — 50 000 units.

- Give test dose and observe for a reaction.

Note It is far easier to insert the nasogastric tube *on admission*, as paroxysms usually become more severe for some days before they improve. Before the initial sedation talk to the child. This is not a neonate but a frightened child having painful paroxysms. Explain what is happening at least initially before he or she is heavily sedated.

Maintain constant supervision
Bed should be near the nurses' station.
- **Chart** frequency and length of spasms as a guide to management.
- **Maintain airway** — have suction and resuscitation tray to hand. If spasms are severe or frequent and prolonged tracheostomy may be considered.
- **Check bladder** daily — and apply suprapubic pressure if necessary to empty the bladder.

Nutrition and fluid intake
Give through nasogastric tube. The child soon goes into electrolyte imbalance if intravenous fluids are continued for days.

Daily assessment
This is essential.
- The number and severity of the spasms are a guide either to increase or decrease the sedation. The *tone*, especially of the abdominal muscles, is also a guide.
- A rapid pulse may be the first sign of infection — or of aspiration pneumonia.

When spasms cease
- Continue to observe carefully during and just after feeding. Regurgitation and aspiration are not uncommon at this relatively late stage.

64

- Encourage to sit up and to do active and passive movements.
- If possible get a lateral X-ray of the spine. A surprising number of children have a fracture.

Prevention

Neonates
- Plan that antenatal women receive 2 doses of tetanus toxoid.
- Work with traditional midwives so they:
- encourage their clients to receive tetanus toxoid;
- learn the value of cleanliness and how to prevent tetanus.

Others
- Tetanus toxoid. Plan for infants to receive D.P.T. 3 doses at monthly intervals commencing at 6 weeks.
- Treatment of wounds.
- Clean all wounds well.
- If previously immunised give tetanus toxoid booster 0.5 ml intramuscularly.

If not previously immunised
- Clean wounds:
- triplopen intramuscularly;
- tetanus toxoid 1 ml subcutaneously and arrange 2 further doses at monthly intervals.
- Deep, dirty wounds or if there is a delay in treatment:
- clean wound well − debride;
- give tetanus toxoid − as above;
- penicillin G and triplopen;
- A.T.S. 1 500−3 000 units intramuscularly.

CHAPTER 4

Diarrhoea

- **Defined** usually as the passing of loose frequent stools, or the passing of 4 or more stools of altered consistency in 24 hours.
- **Commonest** from the age of 6–18 months when many babies are being weaned.

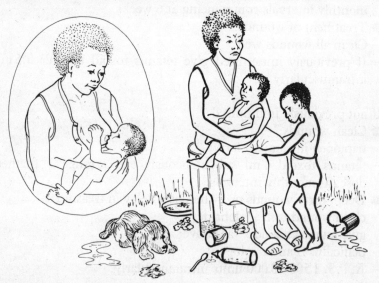

Hazards in the weaning period

Tradition and the facts

It has been the tradition in many places to treat diarrhoea with sulfas or other antibiotics. This has been handed down from senior staff to new staff. The mother is happy with the 'medicine' and the one treating is happy that she has given the mother what she expected and wanted.

But are we facing the facts? Some facts are well known but others came to light more recently. We must face them and act on them.

Table 4.1

Facts in brief	Action
● Diarrhoea is the *commonest* cause of children's death in developing countries. Death is due to loss of much water and salts in the stools causing **dehydration**.	Replacing water and salt is the most *urgent* and *important* treatment. Mothers should be taught how to do it, so as to start rehydration at home.
● **Oral rehydration**, given correctly, will rehydrate *almost all* those dehydrated. It works! This is because the *glucose* released by the digestion of *sugar* present in the water *helps* the body to absorb the salt and water.	Intravenous fluids are only necessary for a small minority of children who are in shock. Have facilities in ward to *teach everyone* oral rehydration.
● Now that the *causes* of diarrhoea are better known, it is realised that sulfas and antibiotics **do not help** the majority of cases. Diarrhoea is often due to a virus, therefore antibiotics are *useless* − of those cases which are due to bacteria, many are resistant to sulfas and some other antibiotics. Other useless drugs are kaolin and pectin − some such as opium, diphenoxylate and enterovioform are *dangerous*.	We must take greater responsibility when treating diarrhoea. Remember antibiotics themselves can be harmful, may *cause* diarrhoea, and give rise to spread of resistant organisms.

67

Table 4.1 *(contd.)*

Facts in brief	Action
● Diarrhoea commonly results in weight loss and **malnutrition**. This reduces the body's *resistance to infections*.	Malnutrition must be remembered — and prevented by: — continuing breast feeding (if breast fed); — giving extra feeds during *and* after the attack of diarrhoea.

Main causes

● **Malnutrition** is an underlying cause (as well as following on from diarrhoea!) When breast feeding is reduced or stopped, not only does the baby lose the food value but also the antibodies in the mother's milk. Diarrhoea occurs more often and is more serious in the malnourished child.

● **Infection** — particularly from contaminated water, feeding bottles, utensils and food which has been standing 'left over' from a previous meal.

Common organisms
● Under 2 years
— More than 50% due to a virus — rotavirus.
  About 25% due to *E. coli.*
  The rest are due to other causes.
● Over 2 years
— *E. coli.* are found in about 60%.
  About 6% due to cholera in endemic areas.
  The rest — other causes.
● Bacillary dysentary — shigella
— is found only in a small percentage of the rest.

Purges and **enemas** are traditionally given to small children in some areas, either frequently as preventive measures or for any mild symptoms.

Clinical possibilities

- **Malnutrition** and **measles** are commonly associated with diarrhoea − it is part of these two illnesses.
- **If fever** − remember malaria in a small child is often associated with loose stools.
- Is there early measles? − check for Koplik spots.
- **If a sudden onset** of very watery diarrhoea and *shock* − remember cholera − see page 92.
- **If blood in stool** − remember intussusception.
- Children with this often end up in the diarrhoea ward!
- The history is of attacks of *sudden pain* and the legs are drawn up.
- Feel for a mass in the abdomen − if the child is resisting, give paraldehyde 1 ml for each 5 kg − I.M. and wait for 20 minutes to examine. A sausage-shaped mass in the abdomen confirms the diagnosis.
- **If there is blood and mucus in the stool** − think of bacillary or amoebic dysentery.
- **If recurrent or persistent diarrhoea**
- Is mother *still* using feeding bottle (infected)?
- Is *someone* in the family still giving strong purgatives?
- Has the child had more than 5−6 days of *antibiotics* − this also can *cause* diarrhoea?
- Giardia infection with frothy stools, heavy strongyloides infestation, amoebiasis and trichuris, are other causes of persistent diarrhoea.
- Lactose intolerance (often a temporary state). Diagnose by finding a reducing substance (sugar) in stool with low pH (<6).

Diagnosis

In out patients

- When many mothers are waiting to be seen, have a person experienced in recognising dehydration walk along looking at the babies. Have facilities ready in O.P.D. for giving oral rehydration salt solution (O.R.S). Mothers of babies with diarrhoea can be shown how to give it, and actually *give it* while waiting to be seen.

● Those with severe dehydration should be sent for treatment as an emergency — in the few cases where intravenous (I.V.) fluids are considered essential, start them before doing the full assessment. Then the fluids are reaching the baby during the history taking, physical examination and decision-making about detailed treatment.

Note It *is* worthwhile to go through a detailed history when first seeing the child — you will probably find the root cause and prevent more visits. So many people say 'There isn't time, I just go ahead and give sulfas! This attitude is dangerous.

History

Use few words — get important facts.
● Stools.
Loose? Watery? Blood? Mucus?
...times a day for...days?
● Vomiting? If yes...times a day for...days?
● Urine: Amount changed? When passed last?
● Breast feeding: Yes/no If no — stopped recently?
● Bottle feeding: Yes/no If yes — what given — too much — how often? What else given?
● Is child drinking to-day? Is child thirsty?
● Food: Pepper? Who gives it?
● Purge or enema? How often?
● Anything else?

Physical examination

Temperature. Pulse. Respiration. Weight.
● Usual general examination. Is the child really 'ill' or not?
● Signs of measles?
● State of nutrition?
● Check tissue elasticity.

Testing for skin elasticity

Table 4.2

		Mild	Moderate	Severe
● From history	Diarrhoea	Less than 4 liquid stools/day.	4–10 liquid stools/day.	More than 10 stools or much blood and mucus.
	Vomiting	None or small amount.	Some.	Very frequent.
	Thirst	Normal.	More than normal.	Unable to drink.
	Urine	Normal.	Small amount, dark.	No urine for 6 hours.
	Condition	Well, alert.	Unwell, sleepy or irritable.	Very sleepy, floppy, unconscious or having fits.
● Look	Eyes	Normal.	Sunken.	Very dry and sunken.
	Breathing	Normal.	Faster than normal.	Very fast and deep, may be 'blowing'.
● Feel	Skin	Pinch-goes back quickly.	Pinch-goes back slowly.	Pinch-goes back very slowly.
	Pulse	Normal.	Faster than normal.	Very fast, weak or cannot be felt.
	Fontanelle (in infants)	Normal.	Sunken.	Very sunken.

Management

Table 4.3

	Mild	Moderate	Severe
● Decide	No dehydration. Use Plan A.	If 2 or more of the above signs there is dehydration. Use Plan B.	If 2 or more of the above **danger signs, there is severe dehydration Use Plan C.**

- Pick up skin of abdomen — hold.
- Let go quickly — if hydrated it springs back.
- If dehydrated it falls slowly back into place.
- Assessment of dehydration — is it severe?

Maintaining adequate hydration is of vital importance. Many children have actually become dehydrated while waiting to be 'seen' or waiting for investigation, so maintaining hydration should commence *before* investigation.

Treatment Plan A

Tell the mother
● She has done well to bring the child before he or she got very sick.
● **To continue feeding the child.**
● Breast milk and liquids (e.g. rice water, juices, weak tea, coconut water) in more than normal amounts.
● If the child is not breast fed and is used to drinking milk, give it diluted with an equal part of cooled boiled water.
● If the child is 4 months or over also give other easily digestible local foods.
● **To watch for the signs** of dehydration, that you have asked, looked and felt for. Show her again how to do this. Ask her to *show you* how she will do this, to be sure she understands.
If the signs come she should come to see you again quickly. Show her how to make up sugar-salt solution and how to give it if signs of dehydration come when it is difficult for her to travel to the clinic or hospital. She should then bring the child as soon as it *is* possible.
● About ways to prevent diarrhoea — (see page 80).

Treatment Plan B

These children are often seen in the clinic and *may* be treated and observed as 'day cases' as long as the clinic staff have the facilities.
There is some dehydration — so water and salt must be replaced.
● If you teach a mother how to make sugar-salt solution and she takes it in — you have taught her for life and she can teach others *at home*.

72

Preparing sugar-salt solution
● Wash your hands.
● Using a clean pot, add 1 litre of boiled cooled water. Find out what local containers equal 1 litre or a little more − e.g. in some areas 3 local soft drink bottles equal one litre − or use 5 × 200 ml cups.
● Add 1 level teaspoon of salt (small spoon holding 4−5 ml).
● Add 8 level teaspoons of sugar and stir very well.
Or
● Using the plastic spoon, add 1 large scoopful of sugar and 1 small scoopful of salt to 1 glass of water. Stir well.

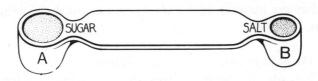

TALC spoon

● Give 1 glassful of the solution for every diarrhoeal episode in the day.

Preparing from O.R.S. packets
These are an alternative, but if in short supply are best kept for more dehydrated or seriously ill children. Packets contain:
− Sodium chloride   3.5 g;
− Sodium bicarbonate   2.5 g;
− Potassium chloride   1.5 g;
− Glucose   20.0 g.
● Wash your hands.
● Using a clean pot, measure 1 litre of clean drinking water (boiled cooled water) using local measures.
● Add one packet of O.R.S. and mix well.
● Ask the mother to taste the O.R.S. solution so she knows what it tastes like.
● Fresh O.R.S. solution should be made up each day and kept in a covered container.

Decide on amount of O.R.S. required for first 4 hours
● If unable to weigh the child, estimate the weight.

Table 4.4

Weight in kg	ml	200 ml cup
3—6	200—400	1—2
7—9	400—600	2—3
10—13	600—800	3—4
14—20	800—1000	4—5

● In older children, *thirst* is the best guide to treatment of dehydration — they should drink as much O.R.S. as they wish. Plain water and other fluids should also be available for them to drink. They should start eating a normal diet as soon as they are hungry; they should not wait for the diarrhoea to stop.

Show the mother how to give the solution

● With a cup and spoon if a baby and from a cup if older. Give a little at a time and watch her start.
● If the baby is breast fed and wants to suck encourage the mother to offer her breast. If the baby is thirsty and wants *more* O.R.S. solution within this time, show the mother where to get more.
● After $\frac{1}{2}$ hour check that the child is drinking.
● If mother says the child is refusing, try yourself.
● If child is refusing to take orally, give O.R.S. by nasogastric drip.
● Even if vomiting a little, fluid is still entering the baby. Continue small sips.
● If vomiting larger amounts and persistently (maybe due to home remedies), give promethazine (0.5 mg/kg) *once* orally and continue fluids orally after a few minutes.
● After 4—6 hours reassess the signs of dehydration.

Re-assessment

● **If signs of dehydration not gone** but child is drinking well, continue Plan B. Give a cup of plain water then give the same amount of O.R.S. solution again for the next 4 hours. Continue breast feeding.
● **If the signs of dehydration have gone,** allow to return home. Make sure the mother knows how to make up O.R.S.

solution by getting her to make it in the clinic. Make sure she has salt and sugar at home.

Advise her to do the following things.

– Give O.R.S.

Table 4.5

Each day	Cups 200 ml
Up to 4 kg	1–2
4–6 kg	2–3
7–9 kg	3
10–12 kg	4
13–14 kg	5

– *Also* give *breast milk* (if breast fed) and other drinks the child likes – e.g. weak tea, orange juice, coconut water.
– If over 4 months old *start feeding* the child 5–6 times a day until well.
  Then give one extra meal a day for a week.
– To *bring child back* quickly:
  1 if the signs of dehydration come back;
  2 if diarrhoea continues and child refuses O.R.S.
– In any case come back in 3 days if diarrhoea continues.
● **If the signs of dehydration are worse**, go to Treatment Plan C.

Treatment Plan C – Severe dehydration

Routes

Fluids can be given intravenously, by nasogastric tube or orally.
● Intravenously, especially if child is in shock. Give fluids orally also if child is able to drink.
● By nasogastric tube if you have no facilities for intravenous treatment.
● Orally if:
– you have no facilities for giving I.V. fluids and referral not possible;
– the child is drinking well and not vomiting;
– the mother is good at giving oral fluids;
– experienced staff able to assess whether a child is improving or not, *and* have the time and the will to make the assessment.

● Later refer the child for intravenous treatment as soon as possible continuing to give the water-sugar-salt (O.R.S:) solution in transit.

Intravenous fluids used
First 24 hours
● **Best all round fluid** − $\frac{1}{2}$ strength Darrows in 2.5% dextrose water. That is equal parts of Darrows and 5% dextrose water. It is best to keep to one fluid and know how to use it.
● **If unobtainable** − Ringer's Lactate (Hartmann's) good initially. It contains adequate sodium and potassium. The lactate yields bicarbonate.
● **If Darrows and Hartmann's unobtainable** − use half strength saline in dextrose water
● **If neonate** − use O.R.S fluid as above alternating with equal amounts of plain boiled water.
For intravenous therapy use Ringer's solution or Darrows − 1 part e.g. 100 ml in 5% dextrose water − 4 parts e.g. 400 ml, for first 24 hours.
Encourage breast feeding.

Guidelines for rehydration therapy for severe dehydration

Table 4.6

Age group	Type of fluid	Amount of fluid (per kg body weight)	Time of administration
	I.V. Ringer's Lactate	30 ml/kg	Within 1 hour.
	followed by		
Infants (under 12 months)	I.V. Ringer's Lactate	40 ml/kg	Within next 2 hours.
	followed by		
	O.R.S. solution	40 ml/kg	Within next 3 hours.
Other children and adults	I.V. Ringer's Lactate	100 ml/kg	Within 4 hours; initially as fast as possible until radial pulse is easily felt.

For infants the entire 6 hour course should be followed to quickly restore the losses of severe dehydration. Frequent assessments are vital.

Follow up

- *Look* at the child and assess the state of hydration at least hourly. The rate of flow may need to be increased to achieve rehydration or decreased if there is puffiness around the eyes.
- Check the I.V. hourly and record the amount given. A strip of paper stuck to the bottle and marked where the fluid should be each two hours makes this possible.
- Talk with the mother and record the amount of fluid taken, also the number and types of stools and vomits.
- While rehydration therapy restores the body's abnormal losses, the normal daily fluid requirements must also be remembered. After 6 hours
  1 For infants – begin breast feeding;
                             – or give 100 – 200 ml of clean water to the non breast fed infant.
  2 For older children plain water should be available for them to drink in addition to O.R.S. solution.
- After the first 6 hours, **ask, look and feel** for the signs of dehydration.
- If there are no signs follow Plan A.
- If some signs are present but the child is improving, give O.R.S. solution for another 6 hours, see table Plan B.
- If the signs of dehydration are the same or worse intravenous fluids must be continued. Follow up as before and reassess in another 4–6 hours.

Possible investigations

- Blood
- for malaria parasites;
- white blood count – haemoglobin.
- Stool
- microscopic examination for blood – pus – ova – parasites;
- culture;
- if checking for lactose intolerance – confirm by stool pH less than 6 and positive clinitest.

Clinitest

Put 5 drops liquid stool in a tube.

Add 10 drops of water and one clinitest (not clinistix).

A yellow or red colour indicates more than ½% sugar. (+)

● *In larger centres*
- Stool culture.
- Widal test.
- Serum electrolytes in dehydration with complications.

Drugs

● In majority give fluids, maintain hydration and observe.
● Give antimalarial course if in an endemic area.
● If you see blood and mucus in the stool rule out intussusception and consider dysentery (shigellosis) — if the child is in good condition he or she will get better. If the child appears ill or in a poor condition give antibiotics.
- Ampicillin 100 mg/kg/day in divided doses four to five days or trimethroprim 10 mg/sulfa sulpha-methoxazole 50 mg/kg/day in 2 doses a day for five days.
- Tetracycline could be given only to those over 8 years. Dose 50 mg/kg/day in 4 divided doses for 4 days.
- If resistant to ampicillin and tetracycline then chloramphenicol 50–100 mg/kg/day in divided doses for 5 days (bearing in mind its dangers).
● In neonates or smaller infants *E. coli* enteritis is likely. Neomycin 25 mg/kg/day in 2 divided doses 4–5 days orally. Consider septicaemia if the baby appears 'ill' out of proportion to the diarrhoea, with a very fast pulse and refusing to suck. Then give antibiotics such as ampicillin.
● If persistent diarrhoea and cause not known, give a course of metronidazole.
- This is also the drug of choice for giardiasis and amoebiasis. If strongyloides or heavy trichuris infestation, give thiabendazole, 25 mg/kg/day in 2 doses for 2 days.
● If lactose intolerance, stop milk for a few days and give more of other foods — Reintroduce milk slowly.
● Treat associated conditions.
● If mother is worried because child is 'only' getting O.R.S.

solution or I.V. fluids – tell her this *is* the medicine for this condition.

Keep mother busy
– watching the drip;
– giving oral fluids and later feeds;
– making sure staff see and describe stools.

Diet

● Breast feeding – Encourage mothers to continue breast feeding as the tradition of stopping food may cause her to stop. Remember **feeding bottles** are often the cause of the diarrhoea in infants who are not breast fed. Change over to cup or cup and spoon.
● In older children and infants not breast fed, continue with the usual diet and diluted cow's milk if available.
● Food – encourage the mother to give easily digestible foods – about 5 or 6 times in 24 hours. (This may also be against the local tradition.)

Talking with the mother, father and family

After assessment and the decision about treatment is made, talk to the mother about *her child*.
● If malnutrition is the underlying cause of the diarrhoea, discuss with her the possible causes and seek a solution.
● If she is using a feeding bottle, explain the dangers.
● If she is giving purges and enemas, discuss this.
● If giving the baby the food prepared for adults with a lot of pepper in it, suggest separating out the child's food before pepper is added.

During your contact with the family, impart to them the following good news.
● Mothers can prevent dehydration by giving *more* breast milk, water and other drinks than normal as soon as the diarrhoea starts.
● Mothers can treat dehydration by giving **oral rehydration salts** (O.R.S.) solution as soon as the dehydration starts.

79

Daily assessment if admitted

Teach your staff to check quickly and report each morning at ward rounds.
● Number of stools in *24 hours* and character − chart.
● Vomiting?
● State of hydration.
● Appetite   Ate anything?   What?
● Weight chart.
If you have these facts you will know what to do next.

Prevention of diarrhoea

● Main factor − adequate water supply to all houses.
● Then − sanitation;
           − health and nutrition education.

Health talk

Convince mothers that death from diarrhoea *need* not happen. Here are 9 points to talk about.

Cleanliness
● Wash your hands before touching food when cooking.
● Wash your hands and child's hands before eating.
● Wash hands after going to latrine. Don't clean up baby's stools then feed baby without washing hands.
● Use cup and spoon − don't hand feed baby.
● Keep food and water covered so flies cannot reach them. (They cause diarrhoea.)

Feeding
● Babies who are fit and strong don't get diarrhoea.
● Keep baby fit by:
− breast feeding alone for first 5 months **without using feeding bottle**, even though people show you lovely pictures of babies with feeding bottles; even though everyone around has one; even though a nursemaid could feed a baby with it while you go to market. (She could also use a cup and spoon.)
● Children are dying as a result of diarrhoea because of feeding

bottles. Why do they sell them then? Because the people who make dried milk want to *sell that too*.
● **When baby is 5 months old start other foods** by cup and spoon. There is danger when *food is left standing* some time, even if covered. − Try to prepare the food fresh for the infant and small child.

Pepper
● Gives babies pain in the belly and often causes loose stools **so cook separately** for the baby without pepper. But that is so much trouble! Not as much trouble as losing the baby, and being pregnant again − and in labour again!

Purges, enemas, home treatments
Babies are dying every day through loss of water from the body, due to purges and enemas. God made trees with fruits and all kinds of vegetables and green leaves. Give baby some of these every day after 6−7 months for healthy movements of the bowel.

Latrine
● Teach your child how to use the latrine − and not to pass stool in the bush or stream. If everyone used the latrine there would be no more **cholera**.

To prevent measles
● We will tell you where to go to get vaccination for the baby.

If diarrhoea starts
You can deal with it.
● Make special mixture:
   salt 1 level teaspoon;
   sugar 8 level teaspoons;
   water 1 litre.
   (Show mother container which holds 1 litre.)
   Give the baby every hour with cup and spoon.
● Stop others giving purges and enemas.
● Most babies will get better with this − but occasionally a baby refuses it or has high fever. If so, go to the clinic and see nurse there.

But you say my mother and grandmother had purges and all these things and they were all right.
But we say to them 'How many brothers and sisters died of diarrhoea?'

Preventing diarrhoea by

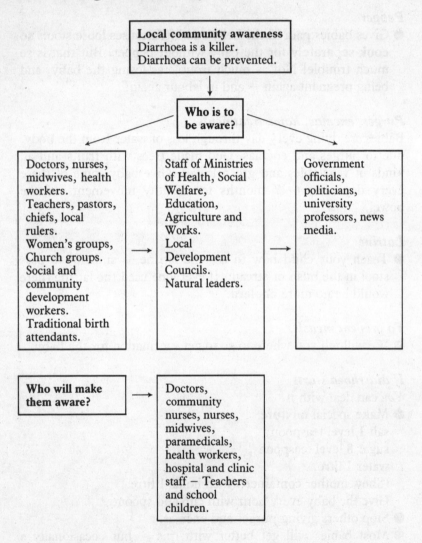

Local community awareness
Diarrhoea is a killer.
Diarrhoea can be prevented.

Who is to be aware?

Doctors, nurses, midwives, health workers.
Teachers, pastors, chiefs, local rulers.
Women's groups, Church groups.
Social and community development workers.
Traditional birth attendants.

Staff of Ministries of Health, Social Welfare, Education, Agriculture and Works.
Local Development Councils.
Natural leaders.

Government officials, politicians, university professors, news media.

Who will make them aware?

Doctors, community nurses, nurses, midwives, paramedicals, health workers, hospital and clinic staff – Teachers and school children.

| How will they do it? | → | Personal example – Person to person talking.
Talking to groups.
Writing articles for local paper.
Speaking at meetings.
Keeping records and getting facts.
Training people in villages.
Lectures and discussion groups with students and nurses.
Communicating with the community. |

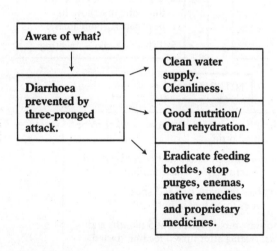

Aware of what?		
↓		
Diarrhoea prevented by three-pronged attack.	→	Clean water supply. Cleanliness.
	→	Good nutrition/ Oral rehydration.
	→	Eradicate feeding bottles, stop purges, enemas, native remedies and proprietary medicines.

What action?

Cleanliness

1 Start where you can and clean individual compound.

2 Aim to get pipe-born water to village and compounds. Married nurses' husbands usually educated and could press for this.

3 Proper excreta and refuse disposal. Keep on and on pressing for it.

4 Newspaper articles and pictures very impressive.

Stop purges, enemas

1 Tell mothers about the dangers of above and also of some native preparations.

2 Give her something *to do* instead:
get immunisations;
get child weighed regularly;
keep weight chart;
dietary advice.

3 Discussions about these with nursing and paramedical students.

4 Write up stories of deaths following diarrhoea for newspaper. (No names.)

5 Talks on radio − meetings.

NUTRITION

1 No nurse, health worker or education worker to be seen with feeding bottle.

2 Hospital staff to refuse posters that advertise dried milks, and even refuse *gifts* of dried milk.

3 Motherless babies fed with cup and spoon. No feeding bottles to be *seen* in hospital.

4 Education to start mixed feeding at 5 months and *continue breast feeding* after mixed feeding started.

5 Start other food at 5 months especially energy foods like red palm oil, groundnuts, soya beans etc. Teach by demonstrations and sharing as well as by talking.

6 All children to have **weight chart**, and attend clinic regularly.

7 Start **nutrition rehabilitation centres**.

8 Train **nutrition workers**.

9 Teach nutrition by songs.

10 Teach and promote oral rehydration.

Government involvement

Concerns several ministries and departments and there would be overlapping of responsibilities.
Following are some of the areas for involvement.

Adequate nutrition
Close liaison between
- Departments of Health
  - paediatric advisers;
  - practical nutritionists.
- Agriculture − to promote the growing of high protein foods by *small* farmers.
- Education − to disseminate information and also Departments of Social Welfare, Development, Transport.
- National Women's Organisation.
- **Advertising** the danger of feeding bottles to the same extent as the baby food companies advertise their dried milk (and indirectly the feeding bottle to put it into).
- **Forbid import** of feeding bottles.
- **Prohibit** local plastic factories to make them.

Cleanliness and hygiene

- Liaison between Ministries of Health, Town Planning, Works, Education, Development and Social Welfare − to succeed in establishing:
  - pipe-borne water to villages and later to compounds;
  - satisfactory rubbish and excreta disposal.

Training health workers
- of all categories − but especially those who will come from and work at village level, and in less favoured urban areas.

Health education
- as part of *life education* through school programmes, health workers, news media − local groups.

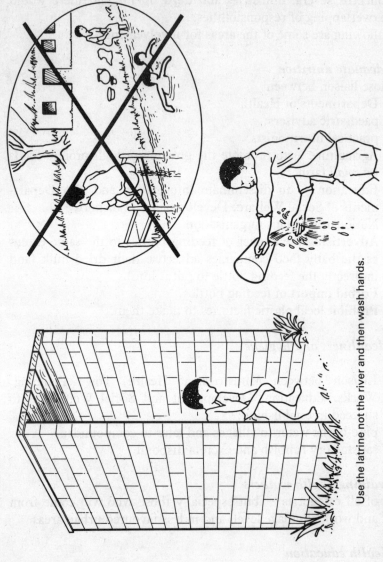

Use the latrine not the river and then wash hands.

Health education as part of life education

Aid to diagnosis – diarrhoea

Table 4.7

Clinical	Possible cause	Associated with	Investigate	Treat
1 Chronic or recurrent (Diarrhoea and malnutrition)	Weaning diarrhoea	Recent cessation of breast feeding. Bottle feeding. Inadequate diet. Poor hygiene. Age 6 months – 2 years. Very common.	History important. Good physical examination. Stool microscopy (usually no pus or blood).	Rehydrate if necessary. If breast feeding, continue. If bottle used – **stop.** High energy infant foods. Long follow up. Educate.
	Lactose intolerance	Insufficient enzyme **lactase**. May *follow* diarrhoea due to other cause.	Stool ● reducing substance? ● acidity.	Stop giving milk for a short time. Give other infant foods high in energy and protein.
	Amoebic dysentery	Low standard of living. Not usually in breast fed. Amoebic hepatitis or liver abscess may follow.	If *acute* diarrhoea check fresh stool for amoebae. If in *remission* check for amoebic cysts.	If in doubt treat with **metronidazole.**

Table 4.7 (*contd.*)

Clinical	Possible cause	Associated with	Investigate	Treat
	Giardia lamblia	Loose fatty frothy stools. Occurs when children overcrowded.	Stool microscopy. One-celled protozoa seen.	Mepacrine (cheap) or **Metronidazole.**
	Associated with kwashiorkor	Poor diet. *Usually not* infective, will improve with good diet over 10–14 days. Occasionally infection also present.	Expect increase in diarrhoea for a few days after starting a good diet, but if does not improve examine stool by microscopy – pus or blood?	● Diet – and expect improvement 10–14 days. ● See chapter on malnutrition.
	Rare: Coeliac disease; Cystic Fibrosis; Inflammatory bowel disease.	Presence of other deficiencies e.g. anaemia, vitamin deficiencies and/ or other constitutional symptoms.	History important. Stool – excess of fat presence of blood and mucus. Presence of anaemia.	Refer for specialist care.
2 Severe dehydration (following diarrhoea)	Any cause or multiple causes.	Any age – less common in breast fed.	After rehydration commenced – careful *history, physical tests.*	Start I.V. *Start – then find cause.*
	Purges and enemas	Cultural belief that they are good.	Ask for details of local medication.	Rehydrate. Observe. Health education.

Clinical	Possible cause	Associated with	Investigate	Treat
	Cholera	Infected water and food. Sudden onset. Rapid dehydration and collapse. '*Rice water*' stools. *Usually* no fever or blood in stools. Unusual in breast fed.	After rehydration commenced: ● look at stool in test tube – rice water? ● rectal swab for culture (if lab. facilities available).	Cholera routine (page 94).
3 Diarrhoea and *fever*	Malaria	Age 4 months onwards. Restless – possibly convulsions.	Blood for parasites.	Chloroquine.
	Typhoid fever	Temperature persists. Diarrhoea may *not be* severe. Child toxic. Spleen palpable. Relatively slow pulse. *Infants* may have infection elsewhere e.g. osteomyelitis.	● Exclude malaria. ● Blood – culture and Widal Test.	Chloramphenicol 50 mg/kg/day (divided) 7 days. Ampicillin same dosage. Nasogastric feeding if no appetite.

Table 4.7 (contd.)

Clinical	Possible cause	Associated with	Investigate	Treat
	Dysentery, bacillary	Abdominal cramps. Mucus in stool and often blood.	Stool microscopy – Pus cells and blood culture.	Sulfadimidine. If resistant ampicillin 5 mg/kg/day (divided) or trimethroprim 10 mg/kg/day.
4 Diarrhoea in infants	E. coli enteritis	*Outbreaks* in nurseries. Malnourished infants, especially those on feeding bottles. High mortality.	If laboratory has facilities to test for pathogenic E. coli – send rectal swab.	● Treat dehydration if present. ● Neomycin 12 mgm/kg. 7–10 days. ● *Some* may be sensitive to ampicillin – 50 mg/kg/day for 5 days or cephalosporin.
		Malnutrition the prime factor – causing low resistance.	Careful weight chart. Blood count. – Stool microscopy. – Exclude other cause e.g. lactose intolerance.	Build up resistance. ● Treat malnutrition. ● Blood transfusion if anaemic.

Clinical	Possible cause	Associated with	Investigate	Treat
5 Diarrhoea with blood	Intussusception	Passage of stools which gradually contain blood and later consist of blood and mucus only (not really diarrhoea but often admitted as diarrhoea). Age 6 months – 3 years. Sudden attacks of pain. Often vomiting. Later – abdominal distension.	● May feel mass in abdomen. ● May feel mass rectally. ● If unsatisfactory examination, give paraldehyde – wait 20 mins. as abdomen will be lax for 10 mins. only.	● Rehydrate. ● Operate.
	Dysentery bacillary	See 3		
6 Diarrhoea with pain and cramps	Purges and enemas	See 2		
	Dysentery bacillary	See 3		

CHAPTER 5

Cholera

The most common world wide form is Vibrio cholera El Tor. It spreads from person to person through hands, bed sheets, other linen or from food which has been handled by a carrier.

It is a self limiting disease if the patient survives 3–5 days, but a small percentage get a severe form and without treatment die of severe dehydration and electrolyte loss.

Clinically

The severity of diarrhoea varies from moderate to severe (classical) with *rapid* dehydration and rice water stools.

Acute onset
● **Diarrhoea** – faecal at first, rice water within hours.
● **Vomiting** early.
● **Cramps** in the abdomen.
● **Dehydration** is rapid with onset of shock.

Severity
● Worse in very old and very young.
● Without treatment or with inadequate treatment, 50% may die.
● With early and adequate treatment, case fatality rate is about 1%.

What happens in cholera?

● Vibrio cholera puts out a toxin (T).
● Toxin passes to lining cells of the gut.

- Toxin acts on an enzyme there which causes:
- water in large quantity;
- sodium, potassium and bicarbonate; to pass into the gut lumen and be evacuated as watery stools.
- Toxin cannot be dislodged from its combination with the lining cells and is active until the cells are shed.

Assessment

Important points
- The period of time from the first symptom or first stool to the time the patient presents. The shorter the time the more severe the attack.
- The degree of dehydration.
- Weakness or collapse – weak patients may *want* to drink but are unable to lift themselves up to hold a cup. They must have a person with them all the time to help them.
- Collapsed patients may benefit from I.V. fluids being pumped in initially.

Why do people with cholera die?

Because of

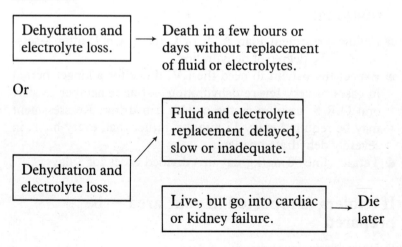

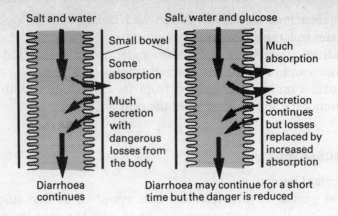

Salt and water	Salt, water and glucose
Small bowel	
Some absorption	Much absorption
Much secretion with dangerous losses from the body	Secretion continues but losses replaced by increased absorption
Diarrhoea continues	Diarrhoea may continue for a short time but the danger is reduced

Replacement of fluids by mouth in acute diarrhoea

Aims of treatment

- **Replace fluid and electrolyte loss:**
- – without delay;
- – in adequate amount;
- – giving needed electrolytes.
- Destroy organism with antibiotics.

Treatment

- Follow Treatment Plan A, B or C (as in Ch.4) after assessment of the degree of dehydration.
- Expect the patient to need the I.V. fluids for a longer period in cases of very severe dehydration – but remember to start oral O.R.S. as soon as the patient can drink. Reassessment may be required every 15 minutes rather than every hour, in severely dehydrated patients.
- Tetracycline 50 mg/kg/day in 4 divided doses for 3 days.

If cholera is reported in your area – be prepared

- Have adequate stocks of:
- – soap, dettol, lysol, tetracycline;
- – O.R.S. packets, I.V. giving sets, Ringer's Lactate;

- alkaline peptone bottles and rectal swabs to take laboratory specimens for initial cases;
- stationery, fluid charts, posters.
● Train personnel in diagnosis and the need and ability to treat rapidly.
● Be prepared to train people to start rehydration centres in the community e.g. in schools or in community centres.
● Be prepared for excreta disposal. Dig latrines if necessary. Have containers with lysol available near them, so this can be poured in them every few hours.
● You will need the cooperation of community leaders – religious leaders, police, politicians, army, and civil servants. Be prepared to talk to them so there is no panic and anxious demands for cholera vaccination for everyone. If cholera is new to your area, try and meet them as soon as the first case appears. Talk about vaccination, health education, and what you are doing to limit any outbreak.

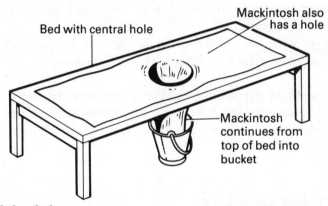

The cholera bed

Vaccination

● Is only 50% effective after 2 injections and a certain amount of time.
● Should not be relied upon as the sole preventive measure because it makes people careless about washing their hands before eating – and this *is* important.
● Many people become cholera carriers following vaccination.

Health education

- **Handwashing** with soap is important. If no soap is available use charcoal, it kills the vibrio.
- **Boil all drinking water** in the initial phase.
- **Chlorinate** all wells in the area if possible.
- Food hygiene – eat food *hot* as the vibrio can live 6–12 hours in cool food. Use *dry* utensils, because vibrios cannot live on a dry surface – but can live 12–24 hours on a wet surface.

To limit the outbreak

- Cases must be treated rapidly. Open several rehydration centres if needed and if resources permit.
- Train auxiliary health workers in rapid diagnosis and treatment.
- Maintain records of what is happening.
- Report and map the number of cases and the area from where they come.
- Those who live in the same households i.e. contacts are offered prophylaxis – tetracycline for 3 days.

Ward staff do not need prophylaxis but must be particularly careful about washing hands and all contaminated clothing. If prophylaxis is given it is easy to become careless and not wash ones hands.

Convalescent phase

Feeding and nutrition rehabilitation important.

Health talk – to patient and relatives on prevention

Cover the following topics.
- A person *can* get cholera a second time. You won't get it if you understand about it.
- Cholera comes from:
- infected water – such as the stream (after someone carrying cholera has washed in it);

- infected food;
- infected stool or clothing.
- Cholera will not be spread via water or food if:
- hands are washed with soap and water after going to the latrine or before eating;
- food and water are kept covered;
- stool is passed in latrine, not on the ground or in the stream. When stool passed in latrine, cover with earth so flies will not carry infection to others.

- If there is cholera in your area, boil water taken from the stream before drinking.
- If anyone in your family starts diarrhoea, give them plenty of drinks.
  Use 1 O.R.S.   salt 1 teaspoon;
  packet to   or   sugar 8 teaspoons;
  1 litre of water,   water 1 litre.
  Bring them to clinic soon if the diarrhoea continues.
- *Cholera vaccine* will not necessarily protect you or your family from getting cholera. It may help somewhat. You still have to pay careful attention to *prevention*.

Note The younger the child, the less likely the vaccine will protect. In older children and adults vaccination may give some protection for 3−6 months.

Cholera ward

Isolation and disinfection technique

Isolation gowns
Must be worn by all staff while on duty in the ward. Clean isolation gowns must be issued each morning.

Masks
Masks are not necessary.

Gloves
- Gloves need not be worn when making beds or doing routine

ward work. They should be worn when in immediate contact with faeces or vomitus, and when sluicing linen.
● Wearing of gloves does *not* eliminate the necessity for washing hands once the gloves are removed.

Hands
● Washed with soap and water (preferably running water), rinsed in Savlon 1%, dried on hand towel.
● It is very important that the water and hand towel are kept clean, so they should be changed by each shift before going off duty and clean water and a clean hand towel left in readiness for the oncoming staff.
● The solution of Savlon 1% should be changed each morning.

Disinfection of soiled linen
Soaked in disinfectants for 1 hour, then sent to the laundry. (Disinfectants like 'Izal', 'Zant' and 'Germolene' produce a 'White fluid' on dilution in water.) For linen use 'White Fluid' in concentration of 1:300.

Disinfection of excreta, i.e. faeces and vomitus
● Should be mixed with an equal quantity of 'White Fluid' 1:150 for one hour before disposal. In practice, 2 pints of W.F. 1:150 is placed in the pail before being placed in position under the patient.
● After disinfection, the excreta is emptied in the trench, covered with clay, the pail rinsed with plain water, fresh disinfectant put in, and returned to the patient.

Dusting, carbolising and mopping of floor
Use a solution of 'White Fluid' 1:600.

On discharge of patient
● Bed, mackintosh and locker mopped with 'White Fluid' 1:300.
● Linen, blanket and mackintoshes soaked in 'White Fluid' 1:300 for 1 hour before washing.
● The bed is then made up with fresh linen, and a pail and emesis bowl left in readiness for the next patient.

Preparation of disinfectants

'White Fluid'

This term covers the disinfectants 'Izal', 'Germolene' and 'Zant'.

W.F. 1:150

- Prepare a pail of W.F. 1:150 by putting 60 ml of pure Izal, Zant or Germolene in a pail (9 litres) of water.
- Use for disinfection of excreta.

W.F. 1:300

- Prepare a pail of W.F. 1:300 by putting 30 ml of pure Izal or Germolene in a pail (9 litres) of water.
- Can also be prepared by mixing equal quantities of W.F. 1:150 and water.
- Use for disinfection of linen, dusting, carbolising and mopping of floor.

Savlon 1% (1:100)

Prepare by using 20 ml pure Savlon in a Winchester bottle (2 litres) of water. Use for rinsing hands.

CHAPTER 6

Measles

Remember five facts

- It's a serious virus disease with a high mortality.
- Age incidence is earlier than in Europe/USA.
- Some clinical features are different from those seen *now* in Europe/USA.
- Severity depends on the state of nutrition and the age of the patient.
- Measles markedly affects the state of nutrition.

Mortality

West Africa – overall   12%.
England – 1960s   0.02%.

Age incidence

West Africa from 5–6 months.
By 1 year one-third of the children are infected.

Clinical features

By the time the prodromal symptoms and fever appear, the virus is firmly established in the body.

Prodromal   *Rash*

T°↗   Coryza   Neck
    → Cough   → Kopliks → Face
Coryza   Conjunctivitis   Body $\xrightarrow[\text{days}]{7-10}$ Desquamates
                                 Limbs

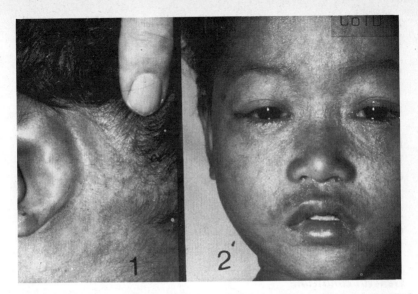

Measles

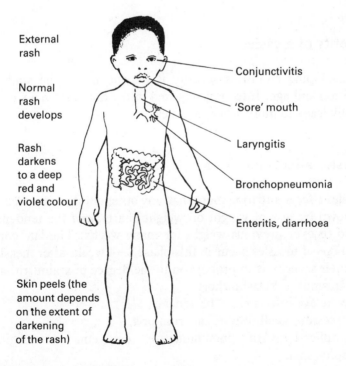

External
rash

Normal
rash
develops

Rash
darkens
to a deep
red and
violet colour

Skin peels (the
amount depends
on the extent of
darkening
of the rash)

Conjunctivitis

'Sore' mouth

Laryngitis

Bronchopneumonia

Enteritis, diarrhoea

Measles affects many organs

101

Manifestations on other epithelial surfaces

Eyes − Conjunctivitis often purulent − possibly corneal ulceration due to associated Vitamin A deficiency. Superimposed herpetic infection is common.

Mouth − Possibly severe inflammation and ulceration. Refusal to drink and eat results in malnutrition.

Larynx − Hoarse − possibly laryngo-tracheo-bronchitis and respiratory obstruction − a danger signal.

Lungs − Pneumonia.

Gut − Epithelial changes causing diarrhoea and resulting in dehydration.

Skin − Desquamates − sometimes in large plaques − leaving oozing surfaces which are easily infected.

General condition

The child may be seriously ill with marked pyrexia and tachycardia.

Severity of measles

In developing countries severity is dependent on the state of nutrition and age. Infection acquired in the home from a sibling usually leads to more severe measles.

Measles affects nutrition

Measles affects nutrition more than any other childhood infection − shown by loss of weight on weight charts, *and* the tendency not to recover previous weight for many weeks. The late complications of measles occur in this phase 2−4 weeks after measles and their severity is in proportion to the degree of malnutrition.

● Marasmus − kwashiorkor.
● Severe eye infections − blindness.
● Abscesses − cellulitis − cancrum oris.
● Complications of pneumonia − empyema − surgical emphysema.
● Rapid progress of primary tuberculosis.

Policy about measles in clinics and hospitals

When a child with measles is seen the possibilities are to:
● treat as an out-patient;
● treat as a 'day' case;
● admit to measles ward;
● admit to general ward.

● **Out-patient** if at all possible − if not seriously ill.
● **Day case** if needs temporary care − e.g. refusing to drink and needs nasogastric fluids for a day *or* hyperpyrexia and in danger of convulsing.
● **Measles ward** if in acute phase (usually 7 days' isolation from the first day of the rash. Probably longer needed for malnourished children) and if any of the following complications is present.
− Respiratory distress.
− Laryngeal obstruction.
− Acutely affected eyes needing frequent care.
− Dehydration.
− Malnutrition (prone to complications).
− Seriously ill in any way.
● **General ward** when child is out of the period of isolation.

In-patient treatment

Routine for all admitted

● Chart weight on under-5 weight chart.
● If under 80th percentile:
− give high energy diet as well as any food the child will take;
− chart food taken on feeding chart.

Child may not wish to eat for 1−2 days when seriously ill − let child have any food he or she *will* eat, at first. Later, talk with the mother about a better diet.
● Fluid intake vitally important − keep chart.
● Haemoglobin or P.C.V. − conjunctivitis masks anaemia.
● Postpone Heaf or other skin test for TB.

Treatment

If fever
- Aspirin 60 mgm/1 year of age − 8 hourly for 1, 2 or 3 days.
- 4 hourly temperature chart.

Fluids
- Check daily on intake − put up nasogastric fluids if refusing.
- Encourage breast feeding mothers to continue.

If pneumonia
- Penicillin, or penicillin and sulfadimidine.

If restless
- Check child is drinking enough.
- Chloral or diazepam (Valium).

Eyes
- Penicillin or sulfacetamide ointment, twice daily.
- 1% Atropine eye drops once daily if corneal ulcer is seen.
- Change to tetracycline ointment if deteriorating on penicillin.
- Vitamin A 100 000 units in water-miscible form by injection daily for 2 days, and orally thereafter for 2 days, if eyes severely affected.

Mouth
- Clean gently twice a day. Good solution is:
  hydrogen peroxide   1 oz ⎫   30 ml ⎫
  normal saline   19 oz ⎭   570 ml ⎭
- Avoid gentian violet because it hides the appearance and tends to dry the mucous membrane.

Ulcerated lips − angular stomatitis
- Often indicates Vitamin B deficiency − give Riboflavin and Vitamin B complex.

Skin
- Wash skin gently − apply calamine lotion − child and mother are then comforted.

If critically ill and toxic

● Hourly or 2-hourly pulse or apex beat and respiration chart.
● I.V. fluids.
● Antibiotics usually given intravenously on the assumption of secondary infection whilst awaiting results of blood culture. Ampiclox best.
● Oxygen if available − when indicated.
● Digoxin if persistent marked tachycardia − e.g. apex beat over 160.

If laryngo-tracheo-bronchitis

● Antibiotic − chloramphenicol or ampicillin.
● Phenergan if sedation required − 1 mgm/kg/dose. Repeat 4−6 hourly.
● Steam tent.
● Prepare for tracheostomy and do early if distressed and not improving or if apex beat and respiration increasing. Better to do an unnecessary tracheostomy than risk a death through being too late. (Always have a tracheostomy pack available.)

Convalescent phase

Dangers

● Secondary infections − watch for and treat.
● Malnutrition − continue stress on good food and discuss with the mother.
● In some areas − Vitamin B deficiency − so give Vitamin B complex and Riboflavin.
● If not improving as should, think of:
− hidden TB − with negative Heaf − treat if in doubt;
− anaemia. Will not respond to iron in presence of measles. If other causes of anaemia treated and child is in poor general condition, a small transfusion (even for moderate anaemia) often results in rapid recovery of general condition.
● Follow up as an out-patient − checking weight chart − diet − and remember to give appointment for *other* immunisations *when fit.*

Risks of mortality continue to remain high for several weeks after recovery.

Priority – prevention

Problems of giving measles vaccine

Maintaining the cold chain
- Europe – plane ⟶ African city airport – still refrigerated. Stored ⟶ transported by lorry ⟶ local clinics and hospital 'fridge ⟶ travelling to outlying clinics.
- This is a challenge to government and ministries.

Often wasted by
- Being given to children who have *had* measles.
- Being given to babies under 6 months who have immunity from mother.
- Residue, after an ampoule opened, being wasted.

Age
The World Health Organisation recommends 9 months. It may not be possible to reach every child in the community at that age and one-third of all children would develop measles before 1 year. However, with regular campaigns of mass immunisation the age incidence of measles is likely to change for the better.

Measles and tuberculosis

If a child already has primary tuberculosis, or tuberculosis in any form, having measles causes it to become more severe. Be sure to continue antituberculosis drugs. If in *doubt* about TB in the presence of measles, *treat* and reassess in 2 months.

● CHAPTER 7

Malaria

Severity

In some parts of tropical Africa 10% of all deaths in children under the age of 3 years are due to malaria. It is especially serious:
● **in children 6–12 months old** because the placentally-derived immunity has faded and the child's own immunity is not yet developed;
● **during pregnancy** – mother's immunity is reduced and she is prone to develop haemolytic anaemia. The placenta is often infected and placental function is compromised, causing poor foetal growth. Clinical malaria in the mother can precipitate pre-term delivery.

Clinically

In children the classical textbook description of rigor, fever and sweating every 2nd or 3rd day is rarely seen. Instead, there are 4 common features.
● **Fever** – irregular – often high or low grade and almost continuous.
● **Convulsions** – usually described as 'febrile'. The seizures may be caused by some 'toxin' acting on the central nervous system in the same way as pyrogens cause rise in temperature.
● **Hepatosplenomegaly** – Splenic enlargement especially is a guide to the incidence and severity of malaria.
● **Anaemia** of a chronic nature with haemoglobin levels of 7–8g is common. With acute attacks superimposed on chronic anaemia the haemoglobin level can drop further and cause acute anaemia with cardiac failure.

These 4 factors are so commonly associated with malaria that wherever you meet one or more you *must* think of malaria first. Remember, checking the blood for malaria parasites is not the answer, as the parasitaemia only remains for a short time.

Typical modes of presentation

Hyperpyrexia

Temperature over 40°C is nearly always due to malaria, which should be excluded first in holoendemic areas. Measles can also cause such a high rise of temperature.

Diarrhoea and vomiting

Associated with high fever is often due to malaria. The stools are liquid, but no pus cells or red blood cells are found.

Cerebral malaria

Due to the blocking of brain capillaries by the infected erythrocytes. Fever is accompanied with delirium, convulsions progressing to stupor, coma and death. Mortality is 25%. There is a high incidence of neurological deficits amongst the survivors.

Blackwater fever

Passing dark urine with increasing anaemia, pallor and prostration. Usually there is a history of administration of quinine. This is not common.

Summary of the effects of malaria

● Death. Mortality is high — especially with falciparum malaria and with clinical presentation of cerebral malaria.
● Repeated attacks resulting in anaemia, splenomegaly, poor appetite, poor weight gain, listlessness.
● Nephrosis reported to be associated with the quartan (P. malariae) form of malaria.

- 'Brain damaged child' following cerebral malaria.
- Increased incidence of premature delivery.
- Low birth weight babies.

Note Children with sickle cell trait i.e. Hb.AS suffer less from severe malaria. In 50 autopsies of children dying from cerebral malaria *none* had Hb.AS.

Treatment

Table 7.1

Presenting picture	Treatment
Fever ● Possible convulsion. ● Palpable spleen. ● Anaemia present and increasing.	● **Chloroquine** *If no vomiting: Tabs 150 mg base* (see dosage table below)

	Age (yrs) Up to 1 yr	1–2	3–5	6–12	13–15
Initial	$\frac{1}{2}$	1	2	2	3–4
After 6 hours	$\frac{1}{2}$	$\frac{3}{4}$	1	1	1–2
Once/day for next 4 days	$\frac{1}{2}$	$\frac{1}{2}$	$\frac{1}{2}$	1	1–2

If vomiting or hyperpyrexia:
Initial dose by injection 5 mg/kg. Then continue as above after 6 hours. May need a second dose by injection.

● **Aspirin**

	Age (yrs) Up to 1 yr	1–3	4–10
mg	75	150	300
tab	$\frac{1}{4}$	$\frac{1}{2}$	1

Repeat 4–6 hourly if temperature still over 103°F (39.4°C) for 2–3 days.

● **To prevent convulsions**
Diazepam 0.25 mg/kg orally 4–6 hourly for 24–36 hours.

Comment
Always exclude other causes. Acute pharyngitis common. Remember urinary infection if fever persists.

Table 7.1 (contd.)

Presenting picture	Treatment
Fever and loose stools (Some authorities believe there is no connection between malaria parasitaemia and loose stools.)	● Treat as above. ● Ensure adequate fluid intake. Fluids by nasogastric tube if necessary. ● Check for *other* causes of loose frequent stools.
Fever, convulsions, semi-coma or coma If persisting: ● brain damage; ● 'cerebral malaria'. **Comment** ● Examine blood for malaria. ● If increased neck resistance or positive head lag test *must* have a lumbar puncture.	● **Chloroquine** 5 mg/kg by injection. Repeat in 6 hours. Some advocate chloroquine intravenously if very ill, but dilute it in 150 ml glucose-saline. Follow up with chloroquine through a nasogastric tube in doses described above. In areas of known chloroquine-resistance, give quinine 5 mg/kg by intramuscular injection. Follow up with oral quinine 60 mg every 12 hours for 6 doses or use Fansidar. ● **Treat convulsions** with *initial* dose of **paraldehyde** (fast and short-acting) 1 ml/5 kg weight by intramuscular injection, and at the same time give a longer acting drug – e.g. diazepam 0.25 mg/kg up to 5 mg. Repeat 6 hourly until improvement, then reduce gradually. ● **Aspirin** As above. ● **Follow up** Inform your senior. Fan or tepid sponge. Keep convulsion and T° chart. Keep child where he can be *seen*. If convulsion has not stopped in 10 minutes, consider more sedation. ● **Maintain fluid intake**.

Presenting picture	Treatment
Collapsed – cold subnormal temperature. No preceding symptoms. Algid malaria.	● **Immediate chloroquine** as above or quinine by slow intravenous injection over 4 hours, diluted in glucose-saline 50–100 mg/100 ml. ● **Take blood** for examination. Malaria? ● I.V. fluid if pulse weak or B.P. low. ● Rule out ingestion of possible poison.
'Passing dark urine'. Blackwater fever. Rare. Have usually had quinine.	● Exclude other causes of 'dark' urine. ● **Never give quinine**. ● Routine antimalarial treatment. In areas of chloroquine resistance, give Fansidar (1 tablet) and inform your senior. ● Keep urine specimens in test-tubes in rack to observe improvement in colour. ● Haemoglobin or P.C.V. 12–14 hourly. ● Anaemia may be sudden and dramatic – needing blood transfusion. Have blood ready.

Notes on dangers of chloroquine
● It is a drug which can cause collapse – if overdose given. So *must* order dose by *weight*, not by age.
● Dangerous if given undiluted intravenously in cerebral malaria, so must dilute in saline 150 ml.
● Can cause death.

Follow up

All Tell mother about prophylaxis.

Dosage of antimalarials for individual protection

Table 7.2

Drug	Dosage in mg according to age						
	Frequency	Infants	1–3 years	4–6 years	7–10 years	11–16 years	Adults
Proguanil (Paludrine)	Daily	25	50	50	75	100	100–200
Chloroquine* (Base)	Weekly	35	75	100	150	225	300

*For areas with known chloroquine resistance, use either Fansidar or Maloprim, or chloroquine weekly *with* proguanil daily.

● Start prophylaxis a week before and continue for one month after being in malarious areas.

If child has had febrile convulsions

Talk to the mother about importance of *preventing* fever.
● Malaria prophylaxis as suitable for the region.
● Give a few chloroquine, aspirin and diazepam tablets and tell her how many to give to the child *in case* fever starts in the night. Then come for check-up.
● If *slight* fever from any cause, come to clinic.

Note Phenobarbitone takes 48 hours to reach effective blood level. Also has effect on behaviour and learning if given long term.

Points to remember
● Parasites are not invariably found in the blood smear because they are transient in blood. Treat if there is any question of malaria.
● If a person is on prophylaxis, one is *less* likely to find parasites in blood.
● Chloroquine is a specific treatment for malaria but correct dose is important. Overdose can cause collapse. Give by *weight* not *age*.

112

- Paraldehyde is the quickest acting drug for convulsions. Know the dose. Give by deep intramuscular injection. Do not use plastic disposable syringe.

Anti-malarial drugs

- Quinine   ⎱
- Chloroquine ⎰ Therapeutic.
- Primaquine – Radically curative.
- Proguanil – Prophylactic.
- Fansidar ⎱ Used where resistant strains. S.E. Asia/
- Maloprim ⎰ S. America/East Africa.

Notes on sulfadoxine 500 mgm/pyrimethamine 25 mgm (Fansidar)
(Combination being used for resistant strains)

Table 7.3

Dose – Treatment	Tabs.	Ml
Adults	2–3	5–7.5
9–14 years	2	5
4–8 years	1	2.5
Under 4	$\frac{1}{2}$	1–1.5

Single dose Do not repeat for 7 days   If injection, deep I.M.

Prophylaxis

Table 7.4

Tablets	Semi-immune Once/4 weeks	Non-immune Once/2 weeks
Adults	2–3	2
9–14 years	2	$1\frac{1}{2}$
4–8 years	1	1
Under 4	$\frac{1}{2}$	$\frac{1}{2}$

Contra-indications Pregnancy – neonates, sulfonamide sensitivity.

CHAPTER 8

Protein Energy Malnutrition

Severe protein energy malnutrition (PEM) shows itself clinically as:

● marasmus − in which the child is emaciated, irritable, and, unless there are complications, has a good appetite;

● kwashiorkor − in which there is oedema, apathy, irritability and poor appetite. The skin and hair become lighter in colour. Cracking and ulceration of the skin − 'flaky paint' dermatosis may follow.

● Marasmic-kwashiorkor is a mixed form.

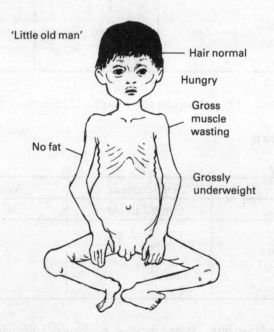

Severe protein energy malnutrition (marasmus)

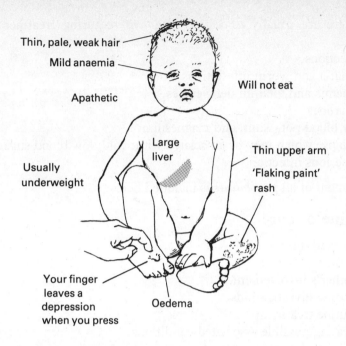

Thin, pale, weak hair

Mild anaemia

Apathetic

Will not eat

Large liver

Usually underweight

Thin upper arm

'Flaking paint' rash

Your finger leaves a depression when you press

Oedema

Severe protein energy malnutrition (kwashiorkor)

Management

Full history and physical examination are vital to establish a thorough assessment of the child's health, state of hydration, dietary and social history.

Principles of treatment

● Severe PEM is a *medical emergency* requiring intensive supervision and care – so treat in hospital if possible.
● The **vital essential factor in treatment** is a **good** and **palatable diet** providing adequate **protein, calories** and other nutrients in a small volume i.e. **high nutrient density**.

The *essential* cause of the condition is *not* vitamin deficiency, *not* folic acid deficiency (although these *may* be also present) but lack of food and precipitating illnesses like diarrhoea, measles or pertussis.

- There are usually *associated conditions* requiring treatment, e.g.
  - infections,
  - malaria and worm infestations,
  - anaemia and vitamin deficiencies,
  - diarrhoea,
  - low blood potassium and magnesium,
  - collapse which may be associated with: cold; low blood sugar; or serious infection.

Treatment of all *possibilities* is included here.

Outline of care

- Diet and fluids.
- Warmth.
- Mother's involvement.
- Routine investigations.
- Routine treatment.
- Treating possible associated conditions.
- Daily assessment.
- Detection of complications.
- Follow up.

Diet and fluids
Correct any dehydration
- If there is any dehydration, which is quite common, rehydrate with oral rehydration solution (O.R.S.). Give by nasogastric tube if the child refuses to drink. If the dehydration is severe, treat with intravenous fluids. Encourage those mothers who are breast feeding their children to continue.

Feeding in the first week
- The aim is to provide some energy and protein without provoking diarrhoea. The strength and volume of the feeds are increased and the number of feeds are decreased gradually in the first few days.

How much?
- For the first 4 or 5 days 125 ml per kg per day. As the appetite returns increase to 150 ml per kg per day, and feed every 4 hours (6 feeds in 24 hours).

Table 8.1

Day	Feed	No. of feeds per day
1, 2	Half strength milk	12
3	Half strength milk	8
4, 5	Full strength milk	8
6 onwards	High energy milk	6

How often?
● Small frequent feeds i.e. every 2 or 3 hours in the first few days reduce the likelihood of hypothermia and hypoglycaemia. Vomiting and diarrhoea are also less likely. Then reduce the number of feeds so they are given 3 hourly − and then 4 hourly.

What feeds?
● Days 1−3 give half strength milk. On day 4 offer full strength milk. In severe kwashiorkor the appetite is unlikely to have returned and nasogastric tube feeding may be necessary for several more days. By days 6−7 high energy milk feed can be started.
● Each child is different. Some may not tolerate an increase in the strength or volume of the feed; in that case return to a more dilute feed or a smaller quantity given more frequently.
● High energy milk diets are based on milk, sugar, and some oil, but some also contain cereals. The oil provides the additional energy necessary for 'catch up' growth.
● As soon as the appetite returns traditional foods should gradually be introduced into the diet so that they eventually replace the high energy milk feeds.
● To prepare the milk and high energy feeds see pages 126−9.

To assess progress and plan treatment
● Keep a feeding chart and record what is offered and how much is taken.
● Record also vomits and stools.
● Weigh and record the weight 3 times a week.
● With high energy feeding most malnourished children recover in 4−6 weeks.

Warmth

Keep warm because of danger of hypothermia and death.
- *Let* the mother hold the child close to her and even take him into her bed — she is a source of heat.
- If the child *has* to be near a window, keep it closed in the cold rainy season.
- Don't go to your warm bed (when the weather is cold) unless you have made sure that the malnourished children have blankets.
- Keep warm and check that you are keeping the child warm by 4 hourly temperature checks.
- **Act quickly** if temperature falls below 98°F.

Mother's involvement

- Establish friendly rapport with the mother and get to know her.
- Obtain information about — the family;

  — their circumstances;

  — their diet.
- Help her to understand the cause of PEM and solve her own particular problem.
- Ideally she should help prepare the food.

Routine investigations

- Complete: Blood count Sickling test Urinalysis Stool for ova/parasites   Tuberculin test
  (**Note** May get false negative.)

Routine treatment

- Vitamins
- Multivitamin syrup 5 ml daily.
- If signs of vitamin deficiency are present, give the appropriate vitamin.
- Oral Vitamin A in oil 200 000 units once (to prevent eye complications).

− Folic acid 5 mgm daily orally.
● Antimalarial − Chloroquine for 4 days in appropriate areas.

Treating associated conditions

●If child has
− **ascariasis** − Piperazine 75 mg/kg daily orally for 2 consecutive days. (Tabs. = 500 mgm Elixir 500 mg/5 ml)
− **hookworm** − Levamisole in a single dose of 2.5 mg/kg or Pyrantel 10 mg/kg body weight to a maximum of 1 g, given orally. Repeat in 24−48 hours.
● If a child is not gaining weight on an adequate dietary intake, then suspect **tuberculosis**. If for any reason TB is suspected, then treat even though the tuberculin test is negative. It *will* be in severe PEM.
● Remember **infections** are common. Check and re-check throat, ears, lungs and urine and treat when necessary.
● If **anaemia**
− Treat any malaria and hookworm present.
− Check for sickle cell anaemia.
− If haemoglobin less than 7 g watch for cardiac failure and treat.
− If *in* cardiac failure because of anaemia, give small transfusion 7−10 ml/kg packed cells with digoxin and diuretic. Repeat if necessary.
− Otherwise diuretics for treating oedema of kwashiorkor are *not* advisable.
● **Desquamation** and **ulceration** may occur in very oedematous feet and legs.
− Clean as for any wound − and dress to prevent cross infection.
− Paraffin gauze dressing (tulle gras) applied to raw areas helps to relieve the pain. When the skin is improved leave off the dressing. At this stage mercurochrome in water is a useful application. The mother can see it and so resists the temptation to apply other things.

Daily assessment and watch for complications

Check and report on
● General appearance and behaviour: Happy? Miserable? Smiling? Engages in play?

- Appetite: Dietary intake? Took what was offered? Needs nasogastric drip? Dehydrated?
- Weight: Unexpected drop?
- Loose stools? Improving or getting worse?
- Temperature last 24 hours — pulse and respiration?
- Unexpected weakness — potassium deficiency?

Detection of complications

Clinically	*Possible causes*
Subnormal temperature 'hypothermia'.	— Insufficient clothing. — 'Silent' infection — septicaemia.
Fever.	— Infection. — Malaria.
Dehydration.	— Insufficient fluid intake. — Diarrhoea. — Did anyone give a diuretic?
Lassitude, drowsiness and collapse.	— Hypothermia. — Low blood sugar — hypoglycaemia. — Infection.
Pulse and respirations increased — enlargement of the liver and oedema.	— Cardiac failure — severe anaemia?

Action

Hypothermia
- Check that the child has sufficient covering.
- Consider severe infection. Examine the child. If septicaemia is being considered take blood for culture if facilities are available.
- Do not delay to treat with broad spectrum antibiotics if you think serious infection is possible.

Diarrhoea
- Possibly an increase in strength or volume was not tolerated.

- Revert for a day or two to a more dilute feed in smaller amounts given more frequently.
- A small number of children have an intolerance to lactose in milk. Stools become copious and watery. If possible test the stool with clinitest for sugar. For this test all stool must be collected on non-absorbent surface e.g. rubber or polythene sheet. If the clinitest is positive and the pH is less than 6, stop the milk in the diet for a short time. Give yoghurt or K-MIX 2 mixture.

Hypoglycaemia
- Do a dextrostix test if it is possible.
- If the child is conscious, give milk or a glucose drink immediately. If unconscious, give intravenously − 50% dextrose 1 ml/kg body weight, or give by nasogastric tube. When conscious give frequent oral feeds.

Infection
- If no cause is found for hypothermia and/or collapse, and if physical examination and urinalysis are normal − presume infection and treat. Gram negative infections are common in severe PEM so use ampicillin or chloramphenicol.

Cardiac failure
- If due to severe anaemia − give a *small* transfusion of packed cells 8−10 ml/kg body weight. Also give digoxin and frusemide.

Follow up

A nutritional rehabilitation centre
This is an ideal half way house from hospital to home. This centre would be away from the *hospital* atmosphere, away from the infections and would cater for:
- children with PEM − now convalescent;
- children with *moderate* malnutrition to prevent it from becoming severe.

If there is no nutrition centre you can help the mother in the ward starting the day she arrives.
- Discuss with her and try to find the specific cause of *this* child's malnutrition.

● Try to show her that this 'sickness' is not due to an evil spirit, or charm or 'bad blood' — show how the child improves on a diet that she can manage at home.
● Talk to *all* the mothers about feeding.
− **Breast milk** is a complete food and it is very important to continue if the child is breast fed.
− A **weaning food** is usually a **basic mix** — that is, a cereal with a protein such as a legume, milk or egg added.
− Later the child will go on to a **multi mix**.
These have 4 basic ingredients. Use local words to name them.

1 **A staple** − the main one − usually a cereal.
2 **Some protein** − such as beans, groundnuts, eggs, fish or meat.
3 **Vitamins and minerals** − a vegetable and/or fruit.
4 **An energy supplement** − fat, oil or sugar.

When these 4 are used together in the right proportions they form a complete meal.

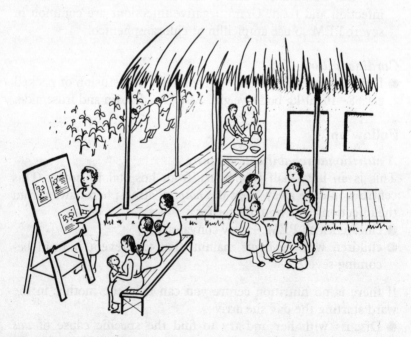

Nutrition rehabilitation

Discharge

- A child is considered fully recovered when he or she reaches the normal weight for the height.
- In theory if the child stays long enough on the above treatment, and weight returns to the optimum, the child goes home and is fine.
- In practice, the mother often declares she has troubles at home and she and the child must go home when the child *begins* to *look* better, but has not yet gained optimum weight. If this is so he can be allowed home:
- when the appetite is good;
- when the oedema (if present) has gone;
- when there *is* a rapid weight gain;
- when the mother understands the importance of continuing the high energy diet at home until full recovery.

Going home instructions

Be specific for this particular child, bearing in mind the child, the mother and the home situation.

- Consider what the child was eating before admission, what the child likes to eat, the financial situation and what food is available — discuss what multi mixes are possible for *this* child, in this place, at this time of the year.
- Talk about weight and weight chart — how you will want to see the child again in 10–14 days.
- If necessary deal with specific cause, e.g. if the grandmother is cooking for the child, make sure you have contact with her too.
- Immunisation appointment if necessary.
- Any special treatment the child may be on.
- Appointment to follow-up clinic or you may have a Nutrition Clinic.
- Tell her she will be welcome to come sooner if worried.

Home visit

If you really want to help this family and prevent severe PEM in later children, it is good to visit the home. Go *with* the mother or else visit when the mother is at home. She will feel free in her own environment to talk about her problems. When you really know her difficulties then you can give advice that is practical *for her* and which she can really carry out.

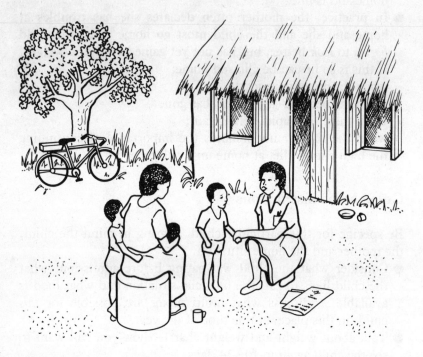

Home visiting

Follow-up clinic

- Weigh the child. Talk about the feeding and assess the child.
- Give further advice and health education.
- Those who are below 80% level of weight-for-age, or those losing weight are '*at risk*'. Duplicate weight cards should be made out and kept in clinic.
- '*At risk*' patients should be seen fortnightly for special care.
- Ideally, those who fail to attend follow up are visited at home.

Further notes on nutrition education in hospital

Who gives this education?

The answer is − *all the staff*. All of them can promote health and good nutrition if they are trained. This includes cleaners, nurses, ward sisters, medical assistants, auxiliaries, doctors and all the staff. Of course, patients soon discover if staff give their own children the good diet they promote in hospital, and they only listen to those who practise what they preach.

What do you need?

● A special kitchen to cook the children's food is the ideal.
● A demonstration area − perhaps the verandah − is good for cooking demonstrations.
● Cooking utensils and facilities similar to the home situation.
● Acceptance by the hospital authorities that this is worthwhile.
● Money to buy the food used in the cooking demonstration. Great enthusiasm and tenacity may be required to obtain all these things − but it is worth the struggle because you are dealing with the basic cause of PEM.

Cooking demonstrations emphasise

● The 4 food types − staple foods, protein, vitamins and minerals, and energy foods.
● Which foods are available and what are the prices.
● Which can be grown at home and the best way to do it.
● How to prepare meals using these foods.
● How to prepare food for those being weaned.

Education also covers:
● the value of breast feeding;
● the dangers of feeding bottles.

Aids to learning are

● Songs about the theme of the day with a chorus that all can sing — they will be catchy and mothers will remember when they go home.
● Leaflets with drawings as well as words.
● Posters if not left hanging up all the time (if they are, they are useless).

What does the community nurse or person concerned do?

● Person to person talks with mothers after general discussions at ward rounds.
● Talking to groups of mothers — daily.
● Explaining their children's weight charts.
● Teaching ideal infant and child feeding, especially about breast feeding.
● Teaching about danger of feeding bottles.
● Showing children who are recovering.
● Cookery demonstrations — daily or 3/week. The mothers may actually cook the food which the children will later eat.
● Discussions about using available protein foods like groundnuts and beans — discuss prices.
● Advice on planting beans, groundnuts and fruit trees.

Ideally   Have an area near the ward with a small **ideal farm**. Get to know the Ministry of Agriculture personnel who will take an interest and give demonstrations. Have seeds to give to the mothers going home.

How to prepare milk feeds

To prepare 1 litre full strength feed
Either fluid milk (boiled and cooled), canned evaporated milk or powdered milk (full or skimmed) can be used.
● Add 50 g sugar (10 teaspoons) to 1000 ml undiluted milk. Goats milk can also be used.

126

- Evaporated milk
  500 ml of evaporated milk is mixed with 500 ml of water and 50 g sugar to prepare about 1 litre full strength milk.
- Full cream powder
  150 g milk powder (30 teaspoons or level scoops) is mixed with 50 g sugar and 1000 ml water.
- Skimmed milk powder
  Mix 75 g (15 teaspoons) skimmed milk powder with 30 g (35 ml) of vegetable oil and 50 g (10 teaspoons) of sugar to a smooth paste. Gradually add 1000 ml of water stirring briskly. If the oil separates on standing, whisk the milk well.

To prepare half strength feeds
- Add 1 litre of water to 1 litre of full strength feed as made above.
- Full strength feeds provide 80 kcal per 100 ml.
- Half strength feeds provide 40 kcal per 100 ml.

Yoghurt preparation
- Mix 50 g (10 teaspoons) of sugar into 1000 ml of yoghurt to make approximately 1 litre.

K-MIX 2
A good mixture distributed by UNICEF for the treatment of PEM.
- Mix 100 g of K-MIX 2 with 50 g (58 ml) of vegetable oil to a smooth paste, gradually add 1 litre of water, stirring well. If the vegetable oil separates on standing, stir briskly before feeding.

Table 8.2

K-MIX 2	Calcium caseinate	3 parts by weight
	Skimmed milk powder	5 parts by weight
	Sucrose	10 parts by weight
	Retinol palmitate 2.75 mg	(5 000 i.u. Vitamin A) per 100 g dry mixture

Preparing 1 litre of high energy feed

Table 8.3

	Milk ml g	Oil ml	Sugar ml
Cow's/goat's milk	900	60	80
*Skimmed milk powder	90	95	75
*Full cream milk powder	120	60	75
*Evaporated milk	430	55	80
*K-MIX reconstituted	130 120	95	40

*After mixing with oil and sugar, make up to 1000 ml with water. Energy value 1350–1360 kcal per 1000 ml fluid.

● If milk powder is being used it saves time to find a 'special measure' to make up 1 litre or 5 litres e.g. if making up 1 litre using skimmed milk powder:
– weigh skimmed milk powder 90 g accurately in the pharmacy;
– find a container which when full just holds that 90 g of skimmed milk;
– label it 'Skimmed milk 90 g' – and use when making up 1 litre of high energy feed.
● Alternatively, tablespoons and cups (250 ml) may be used.

Table 8.4

	Milk	Oil (tbsp)	Sugar (tbsp)
Cow's/goat's milk	3¾ cups	5	7
Skimmed milk powder	13 tbsp	8	7
Full cream milk powder	15 tbsp	5	7
Evaporated milk	1¾ cups	5	6
K-MIX 2 unreconstituted	10 tbsp	8	4

   1 tbsp = 15 ml or 12.5 g sugar
   1 cup = 250 ml or 208 g sugar
   Energy value   1350–1360 kcal per 1000 ml
          or   135–136 kcal per 100 ml

The oil is valuable for 'catch-up' growth. Most vegetable oils can be used.

To prepare
- If using milk powder – mix with sugar and oil to a smooth paste, then add to it small quantities of warm – not *hot* – water that has been boiled and cooled. Mix with an egg beater. If using an electric blender all the ingredients can be blended together.
- If using fluid milk – an electric blender is best, but a rotary egg beater can also be used. Clean the beater or blender very well after each use.
- If a refrigerator is available, prepare feeds for 24 hours and stir vigorously if oil separates. If there is no refrigerator, feeds must be made up every 6 hours.
- If an electric blender is not available, the addition of cereal flour 50 g/1000 ml prevents the oil rising to the top of the prepared feed.

Cow's milk	1000 ml	or	4 cups
Sugar	50 g		4 tablespoons
Cereal flour	50 g		7 tablespoons
Vegetable oil	30 g		4 tablespoons

- Mix sugar, flour and some milk to form a smooth paste. Stir in the rest of the milk. Heat over a low flame, stirring all the time. Boil for 2–3 minutes. Remove from heat and stir in the oil. There are 135 kcal and 3 g of milk protein per 100 ml.

How much?
- 150 ml of high energy feed/kg.
- Give ideally in 6 feeds over 24 hours – in 4 hourly feeds.
- From the third week offer traditional foods, and gradually reduce the high energy feeds.
- **Older children** recovering from severe malnutrition can be given high energy foods with added oil rather than a totally liquid diet.

Nutritious foods

These should be started when appetite returns. Method of cooking and the food available depends on the locality – but here are the possibilities in one locality.

Morning
- Porridge made from maize or other staple with added milk, or pounded groundnuts, or fish cooked in oil.
- Mashed white beans made into a ball and fried.
- Fried plantain or bread.
- Egg if available.

Midday
- Groundnut soup.
- Bean and rice or maize stew or meat and vegetable stew. Use butter or palm oil or any other form of cooking oil. Fish and vegetables with rice. Groundnut stew with meat and vegetables.
- Fresh fruit.

Evening
- Egg if child has not had one already in the morning.
- Softly boiled rice with fish or mincemeat.
- Rice and beans.

Points to consider in preventing recurrence of severe PEM

Typical causes – often multiple	Basic cause	To do – hospital	At clinic
Breast feeding/or milk and cereal only for 10–11 months. Enough food but all starchy. Lack of knowledge that eggs, groundnuts and beans and oil are good for children.	Ignorance. Culture. Tradition.	Nutrition education by person to person and general talks. Cooking demonstration. Cookery participation. Demonstrating children who recovered with proper feeding.	Follow up at Under 5 clinic. Nutrition Clinic.
Parents separated – grandmother feeds child. Can only afford cassava, plantain or cereal. Father 'away' 6 months – money finished.	Parental separation. Poverty.	Community nurse should visit home. If impossible, invite male relatives to hospital and talk. Advise re: planting of beans, groundnuts.	Community nurse to keep in touch. Possibly social welfare may help.
Stopped breast feeding because of another pregnancy.	Another pregnancy within 12–15 months.	Teach responsible parenthood and birth spacing.	Continue teaching at clinics.
Changed from breast to bottle-feeding at 5 months because 'everyone is doing it'.	Stopped breast feeding early. Dilute bottle feeds.	Campaign against bottle feeding. No posters of bottles in hospital. No feeding bottles at all in hospital. Junior staff stop feeding bottles with own children and so set example.	Continue teaching at clinics.
Recurrent diarrhoea for months. Recurrent 'fever' (malaria). Recent measles.	Infection.	Children's clinic. Teach hygiene – cleanliness – use of latrine. Immunise against measles. Campaign against feeding bottles.	

131

CHAPTER 9

Whooping Cough – Pertussis

Important facts to be remembered

● Pertussis is highly infectious.
● Pertussis is a killing disease in small infants.
● Pertussis causes malnutrition and chronic ill-health in many young children.

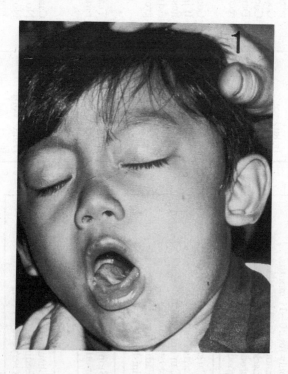

Whooping cough

Pertussis is highly infectious

Therefore:
- treat as out-patients as far as possible so as not to infect susceptible children in the ward;
- if admitted, the child should be isolated alone or with other patients with pertussis.

Isolation required until spasmodic cough and whoop have ceased for 2 weeks, or, if persistent whooping, 4 weeks from onset of spasmodic cough.
- Remember to discharge and treat as out-patient as soon as possible.
- Attack rates in susceptible children in the family may reach 90%. Many of them may be already incubating the illness, so home visiting to check the children in the family and the compound is mandatory. Carry out an immunisation campaign in the neighbourhood.

Pertussis is a killing disease in small infants

Therefore:
- it is advisable to give pertussis immunisation early − at 6 weeks;
- infants in the family who have been in close contact with the patient need to be protected with erythromycin 40 mg/kg/day for 5 days at least. Chloramphenicol 50 mg/kg/day may be used if erythromycin is not available.
- Learn to recognise the disease in the small infant.
- Cough is not unusual at first, but later may be repetitive. **There is usually no 'whoop'** in the small infant.
- Attacks of cyanosis or apnoea may follow what seems to be a slight bout of coughing.
- The tongue often protrudes.
- Sticky mucus may present at the mouth.
- The infant may be brought because of a haemorrhage under the conjunctiva, or an unexplained convulsion.
- If in doubt, ask if other children have whooping cough − it may clinch the diagnosis.

Treatment

- In early stages: erythromycin 40 mg/kg or chloramphenicol palmitate 50 mg/kg/day in divided doses for 5 days. By the time the patient is well into the catarrhal stage or has started to whoop, the antibiotics are of little use.
- If pneumonia also present − give a course of penicillin.
- Teach the mother to handle the child very gently.
- If very ill, may need feeding through a nasogastric tube and frequent removal of viscid mucus from the mouth. Care should be taken to avoid provoking a paroxysm by being very gentle with the sucker.
- If vomiting, give small doses of promethazine 0.5 mg/kg dose.

Pertussis often causes malnutrition

This is because it disrupts feeding and because of paroxysms of cough associated with handling and feeding. Therefore prevent nutritional disturbance by teaching the mother to:

- give energy-rich food in small quantities frequently − not 3 bulky meals a day;
- handle gently before and during feeding;
- re-feed after 20 minutes if he vomits.

Pertussis often causes chronic ill-health

This is due to collapse of a lobe or part of a lobe of the lung followed by chronic infection, and chronic cough.

- Maintain as good a state of nutrition as possible during the acute phase, thus helping patient's resistance.
- Treat with antibiotic if there are clinical signs of infection in the lungs during the acute phase.
- If *whoop* persists in a child, or if coughing continues for more than 2−3 weeks after the acute phase, send for chest X-ray. If collapse is present, the child needs specialist treatment.
- If there is no specialised treatment available, do postural drainage and clapping with cupped hand over appropriate area.*
- Culture the sputum, and give an appropriate antibiotic for 7 days. As infants do not produce sputum, do stomach wash-out with sterile tube and syringe, and send for culture. Ask for *predominant organism*.

- Persistent ill-health and cough in a child who has had whooping cough must raise the suspicion of the activation of a dormant tuberculous focus. Mantoux test may be negative. Follow ups including repeated X-rays may be needed to establish the diagnosis of tuberculosis, but do not delay treatment if tuberculosis is suspected.
- Recurrence of 'whooping' at the next episode of respiratory infection is a frequent occurrence.

*See section on 'postural drainage and clapping' in Chapter 25.

● CHAPTER 10

Tuberculosis

- Tuberculosis is common in persons of all ages and causes much illness and many deaths. In children it tends to be a general disease involving several organs unlike the adult in whom the lungs are most commonly affected.
- Tuberculosis is spread from person to person when anyone with lung tuberculosis coughs and throws out many tiny droplets which carry TB bacteria.
- These small drops can remain hanging in the air, especially inside a room or other place where the air is still. They can then be breathed in by others — children or adults — who then might become infected. Sometimes these drops can settle on to food or liquids which are then given to children. If cattle get tuberculosis their milk can become infected.
- Children can in this way breathe TB bacteria into their lungs or swallow them in their food or drink. The first is much more common than the second but that should not be overlooked.
- When children are infected in this way for the *first* time the bacteria settle and multiply in a lung, in the intestine, or on any surface where they can penetrate. This is known as the *primary focus*. From this point bacteria are carried to the nearest lymph glands which then become enlarged. Depending on the position of the first infection these glands appear at the root of the lung, in the abdomen, in the neck, armpits or groin. Only in the last 3 places are they visible.
- The tuberculous changes at the place of first infection and the glands which go with it are known as the *primary complex*.
- As this complex forms some bacteria escape into the

circulation and are carried to other parts of the body such as brain, bones, liver and spleen.

● About 6−8 weeks after infection a person becomes sensitive to tuberculin − an extract made from TB bacteria − so this can be used as a test for previous infection.

● Most cases heal − slowly over many months − but in some children the infection progresses in the lungs, the lymph glands or in the brain or bones. This is more likely to happen:
− the younger the child at the time of infection;
− the poorer the state of nutrition;
− after measles, whooping cough or other acute infection.

● Complications can be prevented if the first infection is properly treated as soon as it is found, whether or not the child appears ill.

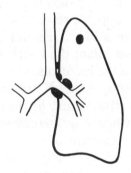

Primary complex focus and reg. glands

Complications

In the lungs
● By continual enlargement of the primary focus.
● In a young child a lymph gland may compress and block a bronchus causing collapse of the lung beyond.
● More commonly a gland erodes through a bronchus, discharging its contents into the bronchus and so causing bronchopneumonia. This spreads rapidly. The slow spread of tuberculosis with much scarring and fibrosis is only seen in older children.

137

In other organs

- Bacilli may be carried to all parts of the body by the blood stream if the primary or its glands erode a blood vessel.
- Spread may be to:
- lungs causing miliary tuberculosis;
- brain causing tuberculous meningitis;
- bones and joints especially spine and hips.

The above are usually within two years after the primary infection.
- Renal and genital infections usually occur more than 5 years after the primary infection.

Clinical picture

Primary tuberculosis

- There may be no obvious symptoms but many children lose their natural energy and appetite so their weight is stationary or falls. They may have a low fever and some cough and wheeze. Sometimes in an infant the cough is like whooping cough due to pressure on the bronchus.
- A positive tuberculin test or chance X-ray finding of enlarged hilar glands or a pleural effusion may be the first hint.
- Think of tuberculosis when a malnourished child does not improve with adequate treatment of some other infection or if the recovery is delayed following measles or whooping cough. When a child is malnourished tuberculin sensitivity may be reduced or lost − then a negative test does not rule out tuberculosis. When in doubt treat and watch the clinical result, especially look for weight gain.

Spread by blood stream

- In **miliary tuberculosis** the child first loses appetite and energy and as the disease advances becomes toxic, feverish and loses weight.
- Cough, if present at all, is usually soft or slight. In the early stages there may not be any abnormal signs in the chest. Later fine moist sounds may be present. Tuberculin test is often negative if the child is malnourished. Under chest

X-ray a fine mottling of the lungs would be apparent.

● **Tuberculous bronchopneumonia** or miliary tuberculosis may be suspected and if X-rays are not available then treat and observe closely. This applies to children with clinical signs of pneumonia, loss of weight or negative tuberculin test, who fail to respond to adequate treatment of bacterial bronchopneumonia.

● **TB meningitis** presents with the usual symptoms of meningitis but over weeks instead of days. Irritability, change of personality and altered behaviour are often the first symptoms. Drowsiness is a late and bad sign. Suspicion is all important. Confirm by lumbar puncture and treat early, for the result of treatment depends on the duration of illness when the treatment begins.

Lesions in bones and joints and elsewhere

These give local symptoms – swelling, pain and alteration of function.

TB glands in the neck

These appear as localised swellings, firm at first and later softening. Signs of redness appear only as the skin becomes involved as the node softens. Pain is not a prominent symptom. Aspiration rather than incision makes local spread less likely.

Abdominal tuberculosis

This often presents as an 'enlarged abdomen' due to fluid. The diagnosis may be suspected if one lives in an area where milk from infected cows is drunk. But remember babies can get abdominal tuberculosis after contact with human infectors. Having excluded other causes of ascites the tuberculin test is helpful.

Investigations

● **Sputum examination** for tubercle bacilli is used in children:
– in suspected tuberculous bronchopneumonia or miliary TB;

- in suspected *secondary* infection in an older child.
  Older children may co-operate to produce sputum. Younger children swallow it so it is best obtained first thing in the morning by gastric suction using a sterile tube. Repeat twice more if negative − but do not delay treatment if, clinically, tuberculosis is suspected.
- **X-ray is a most important investigation** but must be interpreted with care and consideration of the clinical picture. Enlarged hilar glands may be present. Collapse, emphysema, pleural effusion and miliary tuberculosis may be seen.
- **E.S.R.** is raised in many infections and other conditions and a raised rate is not specific for tuberculosis.
- **In summary** the diagnosis may not be easy but a careful history with the picture of vague ill health, a possible contact especially within the family situation and the proper use of the tuberculin test makes it possible.

Management

Principles of treatment

- **The object** of treatment is to:
- sterilise the primary focus and lymph nodes;
- provide cover for the period when the disease is most likely to spread − for at least 12−14 months after infection.
- **Response to treatment** is slow, taking a year to 2 years, therefore ensure the whole course is completed by every means possible.
- The **vital factor** in curing tuberculosis is the **drug treatment**. Studies have shown that the anti-TB drugs are *the vital* requirement although adequate food and treatment of other infections and infestations are both important and must receive attention. It is *unwise* to give unnecessary vitamins and tonics as the family may remember to give these, rely on them, and fail to give the anti-tuberculosis drugs.

Drugs

Make the treatment as cheap, painless and simple as possible. INH and thiacetazone are both cheap and effective drugs. Streptomycin is not necessary for simple primary infections and should be used only when there is acute illness or if other drugs are not available to be given with INH.

Follow up
Discuss with the family and try and get their co-operation. At the hospital decide how to make it possible for you to follow up – either at a special TB clinic, or with special TB treatment cards. In this case the treatment must also be written on the card used in outpatients as this is where the child will probably return.

Anti tuberculosis drugs

First line drugs
- All drugs are taken orally except streptomycin which is by injection.
- All drugs to be given as a single daily dose except P.A.S. may be given 2–3 times a day if it is difficult to take in one dose.

Isoniazid – (INH)
- The most important drug. It is completely absorbed and enters body fluids and cells. It is a cheap, easy to take tablet and in children virtually non-toxic. Most effective in a single morning dose/day.
- **Dose** Prophylaxis 5–10 mg/kg/day orally.
  Treatment 10 mg/kg/day except for the acutely ill then 15–20 mg/kg/day, maximum 400 mg/day.
  Also give pyridoxine 40 mg/day in malnourished children.

Streptomycin sulfate
This is also bactericidal (kills the bacteria) and diffuses into the C.S.F.
- **Dose** Given once daily intramuscularly.
  30 mg/kg from 2 weeks to 1 year.
  At 1 year 250 mg and at 7 years 500 mg.
  At 14 years and above 1 g (maximum dose).
- There are very few toxic reactions by deep I.M. injection. Damage to the 8th nerve is said to occur, but experience has

shown that this is rare in children. Skin sensitivity can develop — so nurses should wear gloves when giving it. Give only short courses, rarely longer than 2−3 weeks.

P.A.S.
● Less effective, but important because when given with streptomycin or INH it prevents the development of resistance and it is cheap.
● P.A.S. can be made in a 25% suspension and flavoured. It will only keep 2 weeks.
● **Dose** 200−250 mg/kg orally, maximum 10 g/day. Give as a single dose or divided 3 times a day.
● **Toxic reactions** Nausea, fever, headache, vomiting, pains in limbs, rash and rarely lymph glands swell. The reactions disappear when the drug is stopped. Miller reports little difficulty with toxic reactions used with INH alone, and rarely with streptomycin *and* INH.

Thiacetazone
● Used as a second drug with INH or streptomycin.
● **Dose** 3−5 mg/kg/day orally.
● Tablets are made combined with INH either:
− thiacetazone 50 mg and INH 100 mg;
− or thiacetazone 50 mg and INH 133 mg.
● These are useful in prophylaxis — but acutely ill children need INH 15−20 mg/kg/day, so give *extra* INH. Use the 100 mg INH tablet. It is important not to give *more* than the basic dose of thiacetazone because side effects, although rare, may be serious.

Second line drugs

The more recent but not necessarily more effective drugs except for rifampicin. They include rifampicin, pyrazinamide, ethionamide and ethambutol. The first line drugs are the basis of treatment. The second line drugs are rarely available consistently in order to complete a course.

Ethambutol
● Not recommended for long term treatment in children.

142

● Enters CSF in meningitis so good in that condition.
Dose 25 mg/kg/day for 8 weeks then 15 mg/kg/day orally.
Maximum daily dose 1 g.
Toxic reactions Gastrointestinal symptoms, joint pains and
toxic eye effects. If eye symptoms occur – STOP drug.

Rifampicin
● Bactericidal – expensive.
● **Dose** 10–15 mg/kg/day maximum 600 mg – give orally
after breakfast.
● Can give with INH, but separate from P.A.S. by 8 hours.
● Do not give long courses.
● Patients' urine, and sputum become red – (not a sign of
toxicity).
● **Toxic effects** on liver function – jaundice – liver enlarges.

Ethionamide
Always give with another drug.
● **Dose** Children under 10 years – 10 mg/kg/day orally and if
no signs of sensitivity 15 mg/kg/day after 2 weeks.
● **Toxic reaction** Sometimes causes nausea and vomiting.
● **Contraindication** Liver disease.

Chemoprophylaxis

This may be INH only. Give to:
● the newborn baby whose mother is sputum positive for
tuberculosis and who will breast feed or be in close contact –
give INH to the baby until the mother has 3 sputum negative
results for tuberculosis. Then give BCG and stop INH which
would kill the BCG mycobacteria.
● tuberculin negative younger children in close unavoidable
daily contact with a sputum positive parent or relative. Give
INH until the contact is sputum negative, then stop INH
and give BCG.

Admission to hospital

This is of no value and there may even be a danger from other
infections except:
● where there are complications – requiring in-patient treatment;

- where there are other illness also requiring hospital treatment;
- where there are social problems in the family;
- if children *need* streptomycin.

Treatment is planned according to the condition of the individual child. The following 3 groups are guidelines.

Group I   Out-patients

- Apparently healthy children who react significantly to the tuberculin test (not having had BCG) in whom the timing of their primary infection is unknown. It has been the custom to treat those under 3 years but now many believe *all* children should have the benefit of treatment.
- Those suspected of tuberculosis, but who have a negative Heaf and associated:
- severe malnutrition;
- failure to improve in the post measles or post whooping cough phase.
  A negative tuberculin test is valueless at this time. The more seriously ill of these would be in Group II.
- In some problem situations of persistent low-grade P.U.O. (pyrexia of unknown origin) when other causes are excluded, starting TB treatment may be diagnostic as there is usually a quick response to treatment.
- Enlarged cervical glands may be due to several causes — tuberculosis could be one of the more common ones in some areas. The enlargement of the glands is slow and painless. Exclude acute infection and blood disease. Heaf test is usually positive. If in doubt, treat. Treat with INH ideally for 18 months — and a second drug — thiacetazone or P.A.S. Treatment may not prevent the softening of the gland, but the aim is to kill tubercle bacilli and to remove the danger of spread by the blood stream.

Group II

- Children with clinical manifestations of tuberculosis, e.g. pleural effusion.

● Tuberculosis of bones and joints. *Refusal to walk* in a child who *has* walked is often the first sign of a tuberculous spine − even before there is a lump or gibbus. A child *limping* should also make one think and check for TB.
● Medical Research Council (MRC) trials show bone disease heals satisfactorily without streptomycin, but 2 drugs, INH, and one other are required. So the child may be treated as an out patient.
● TB pericarditis and pericardial effusion present with fever, malaise and loss of weight. Clinically the pulse is weak and rapid, the heart sounds are faint and the heart and liver are enlarged. Do the tuberculin test. If in doubt whether it is tuberculosis or not − treat.
● Ascites may be due to tuberculosis. The tuberculin test may be positive or negative. Treatment may result in rapid improvement if it is due to TB.

Treatment
● It is essential to give two drugs:
  1 INH;
  2 Thiacetazone or P.A.S. − in sufficient dosage and regularly − for 18 months to 2 years.
● Streptomycin injections may be given − if indicated − until fever settles usually in 2−3 weeks.

Group III   Admitted

● Seriously ill with:
− miliary tuberculosis;
− extensive pulmonary tuberculosis; or
− tuberculous meningitis.
● *Speed* is essential − with the full weight of therapy.
  1 INH 15−20 mg/kg/day orally. A maximum 400 mg/day. If the child is malnourished add tablets pyridoxine 20−40 mg/day.
  2 Rifampicin if available. Streptomycin if not.
  3 Third drug P.A.S., thiacetazone or ethambutol.
● In TB meningitis decide whether or not to give intrathecal streptomycin − 10−50 mg/dose/day for 10 days. This is difficult unless facilities are adequate as other infections may be introduced with repeated lumbar puncture. Corticosteroids

may be given orally if there is cerebral oedema. Try to isolate the organism by culture and do sensitivity. Treat from 18 months to 2 years.
- Sensitivity to treatment and response is noted by the:
  - clinical condition;
  - ability to take fluids and food;
  - weight gain.

Drugs
- Streptomycin is withdrawn after 8–12 weeks.
- If on INH and rifampicin stop rifampicin after 3–4 months or sooner if there is toxicity.
- Then continue INH and a second drug until the treatment is completed.
- Resistance is not such a problem as in adults.

For all groups

Routine
- Full physical examination is essential – looking especially for other possible infections.
- Check haemoglobin and treat anaemia if present.
- Check stool for parasites.

Nutrition
- If an out-patient discuss with the mother about the child's diet. Check and chart the weight at regular intervals.
- If an in-patient see that the child is offered 3 nutritious meals a day, with snacks in between. This requires enthusiasm and good management as there are usually many problems to overcome!

Family check up is essential
- Try and find out from whom the child has caught tuberculosis.
- It is often surprisingly difficult to persuade parents to allow a family check up to be done.
  - Take a history as to *who* is living in the house, including relatives, friends and lodgers, and ask if anyone is sick or has a cough.
  - Make a list on the OPD card. See and examine all children

for TB. Aim also to see and examine any adult whom you think may be infecting others with TB.

Overview of treatment
● Whatever the treatment it is wise to write:
− the drug or drugs ordered;
− the months when the child is expected to return to collect the drugs.
● Otherwise when the child attends OPD for another complaint, it may be overlooked that treatment for TB is also required. In this way one can also see at a glance if the child has failed to return for follow up.
e.g. INH 1/2 tablet daily for one year.

MAR	APR	MAY	JUNE	JULY	AUG	SEP	OCT	NOV	DEC	JAN	FEB

● Give fresh supply every 1−2 months, and tick off when given.

If admitted send home with
● One month's supply of anti-TB drugs.
● Any other treatment necessary.

● Arrange to complete family check up if not finalised.
● Enter into the TB register.
● Write the date of the next appointment on the OPD card and also on the 'Under 5' card − if appropriate.

Community care and prevention

Four things are required to reduce the amount of tuberculosis in any community.
● Find adults with active tuberculosis and treat them adequately.
● Check all contacts of sputum positive adults.
● Use the tuberculin test to find infected children and treat them.
● Give BCG to newborn and tuberculin negative children.

147

Therefore decide in *your* hospital or clinic what you can do — working with others to achieve this.

Community awareness

This is vital, whatever you do, Important facts to get over are as follows.
- Tuberculosis *can* be cured.
- Tuberculosis gets better *quicker* when treatment is started *early*, so do not delay once it is suspected by a persistent cough, or cough and sputum in an adult.
- It *will* take a long time, 12−18 months.
- Patients will *feel better* before they are cured, so they will have to continue taking drugs even after they feel better.
- TB spreads by droplet infection during coughing — it happens especially when someone sleeps in the same room as a TB patient, so if possible let the patient sleep alone.
- If a person is diagnosed as having TB explain about family check up.
- Vaccination of newborns and children with BCG.

- **Who** can provide this community awareness?
- **To which people** or groups?
- **How** will they do it?

Tuberculin testing

Tuberculin testing to estimate the body's antibody reaction to tuberculosis may be carried out by using various tests, the multiple puncture Heaf test and the Mantoux single intradermal injection being the most commonly used. The multiple puncture method is used as a screening test and the intradermal (Mantoux) test in most clinical work.

Heaf test

This is a routine test on admission except for
- Those who have had it done recently.
- Those known to have tuberculosis.
- Neonates (who get BCG without it).
- Those with measles or recent measles.

148

● Those who have a rash, so that it would be impossible to read. (Do later.)

To simplify matters
● Do on the *left forearm*.
● Do on the *inside* where the skin is light.
● Do exactly half way between elbow crease and wrist.
● Mark with small piece of strapping *below* Heaf – (Biro washes off).
● Mark on chart and immunisation card and sign your name and date.
● Read 4–7 days (not 2–3 days) later because some children are *late reactors*.
● If negative arrange BCG in a child who has not had recent measles or is not seriously malnourished.
● If positive ask again and look for previous BCG mark. If none, proceed as for *positive Heaf*.

Remember do not perform the test on neonates – give BCG. Do not do the test in cases of measles or recent measles, but arrange to test in 2 months' time.

Method of performing Heaf test
● Use Heaf multiple puncture apparatus.
● The plates used in the apparatus must be sterile. Ideally they should be autoclaved, but they may be boiled or sterilised by 'flaming'.
● The Heaf 'gun' itself need not be sterile, but must be very clean. It may, and should, be sterilised from time to time. New models may be autoclaved.
● The tuberculin solution used is P.P.D. (purified protein derivative).

Technique
● Cleanse the skin with soap and water.
● When the skin is dry place one drop of the tuberculin solution on to the skin from a sterile syringe and spread to cover an area of about 1 cm.
● If the apparatus has a penetrating depth device, set it at 1 mm penetration for infants under 2 years, and at 2 mm penetration for all others.

149

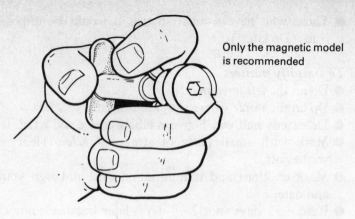

Only the magnetic model is recommended

Heaf apparatus

- Place the end plate of the Heaf 'gun' firmly on the skin in the centre of the film of P.P.D. and tense the skin between a finger and thumb.
- Press the handle of the apparatus. This causes the points to pierce the skin, carrying a small amount of P.P.D. with them.
- Allow to dry. No dressing is applied.
- Care must be taken throughout that no trace of disinfectant is allowed to come in contact with either skin or apparatus. Check that the skin *has* been punctured and in the correct 'wet' area.

Reading the Heaf test
The test may be read from the 4th to the 7th day. The 7th day is best.

Negative reaction
Absence of induration signifies absence of tuberculin sensitivity.
A negative reaction will appear as follows.
- Minute puncture scars without redness.
- Minute puncture scars with slight redness but without any induration, which can be felt by the finger tip.

In a negative reaction, any small punctate spots at the site of the punctures disappear when the skin is stretched.

150

Negative	Increasing degrees of positiveness ──────────►			
0	1	2	3	4
–	+	++	+++	++++
Faint marks No induration	4 or more discrete palpable papules	Papules have coalesced, normal skin inside circle	Normal skin obliterated	Blistering present

Heaf test reading

Positive reaction

Palpable induration of at least 3 puncture points is a positive reaction, but if the test was properly done, there will be 6 such points. The induration is best felt by passing the end of a finger over the punctures.

A positive Heaf test means either:
● the child has had BCG;
● the child has had TB some time – not necessarily active now;
● the child has active TB *now*.

Remember to ask if BCG has been given, and *look* at the particular shoulder which is the site used for BCG in your area.

Note The severity of the reaction depends on the body's ability to react to tuberculin rather than the severity of the infection. BCG rarely causes a grade 4 positive reaction.

Intradermal Mantoux test

● **Use**
– Mantoux 1 ml glass syringe, do not use it for any other purpose.
– Fine needle gauge 26–27.
– Standard test, tuberculin 1:1000 – that is 10 units in 0.1 ml of fluid.

But if Tween 80 is added then P.P.D. 2 units is sufficient. Tween 80 stops the tuberculin sticking to the glass.

Tuberculin should be dissolved with a special diluent. Solutions already diluted are obtainable from the manufacturers but do not retain their potency for long periods. When adding the diluent write the date on the bottle and do not use after 1 month. Store at 2°–10°C. Any material in an *open* phial should be thrown away at the end of a session.

● **Route** Intradermal after washing and drying the skin. Do not swab with spirit or antiseptic. Using the special syringe and fine short needle some resistance is felt at first as the needle enters the superficial layers of the skin and then as the needle enters the correct layers a small weal appears.

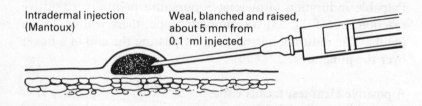

Intradermal injection (Mantoux)

Weal, blanched and raised, about 5 mm from 0.1 ml injected

Mantoux test

● **Reading** Read at 48–96 hours.

If there is an area of redness, with a round raised area of 6 mm or more the test is positive.

This shows the child either:
– has had BCG;
– has had a primary infection which may be healed; or
– has active tuberculosis causing his current illness.

● CHAPTER 11

Poliomyelitis

● Poliomyelitis is caused by a virus of which there are 3 strains. It is transmitted by the oro-fecal route and by person to person contact. After ingestion it is replicated in the alimentary tract and adjacent lymphoid tissue. After spreading to deep lymph nodes it disseminates along the blood stream and reaches the nervous system.

● It affects principally the motor and autonomic neurone cells of the spinal cord, but may affect the base of the brain, chiefly the motor nuclei of the mid-brain.

● Due to polio immunisation, new cases of paralytic polio have become a rarity in Europe and North America during the last fifteen years.

– 3 drops of vaccine on sugar cube taken by mouth.

● In tropical countries, the virus is widespread and the majority of children are infected by the second or third year of life. This can be shown by the presence of antibodies to polio in their blood.

● Only the occasional child develops paralytic polio, but some who do have a crippling disease. Many children are left with weak or paralysed limbs. Usually there is *some* degree of recovery, and even without sustained care many are able to walk. A few of these children eventually become mobile and are able to fend for themselves. Many others die neglected.

● In countries with poor hygiene, babies acquire the infection early when they still have some maternal antibodies, so the infection is mild and not paralytic. As the level of hygiene improves in a country, contact with the polio virus tends to be later, e.g. in the second year onwards, when there is no longer immunity from the mother. Illness then will be more severe and there will be more paralytic polio. This is borne out in Africa where the incidence and severity of polio have increased in the last 10 years and are still increasing.

Main aims in poliomyelitis

Immunise every infant against the infection by mass campaigns.
● In the meantime, treat new cases in hospital.
● Set up simple rehabilitation units to find the handicapped, get them walking and improve the quality of their lives.

But how do these children actually *present* at *hospital*?
Some typical presentations are given here.

Acute illness (Polio?)	'Feverish and miserable and cries when I move her neck — for a few days.'

Acute illness, pain + weakness of limb Spinal polio	'Feverish, miserable — cries when I move her and has one weak leg.'

Weakness of limb Recent acute polio	'Refuses to stand or take steps for last 3 weeks. Yes, she *did* have a fever and had injection at home for it.'

Weakness and contractures Post-polio	'Many months ago she suddenly stopped walking — now she can only sit and crawl.'

Never walked Post-polio?	'And is now aged over 2 years!'

154

Less common

Acute illness and cannot swallow
Bulbar polio

'Has had fever for a few days and now cannot swallow and his voice has changed – Isn't breathing properly.'

High fever for days confused
Polio encephalitis

'The fever just goes on and on and he isn't talking sense.'

Differential diagnosis of poliomyelitis

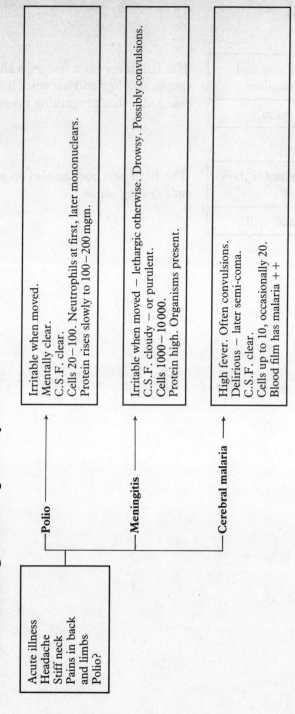

Acute illness
Headache
Stiff neck
Pains in back
and limbs
Polio?

Polio →
Irritable when moved.
Mentally clear.
C.S.F. clear.
Cells 20–100. Neutrophils at first, later mononuclears.
Protein rises slowly to 100–200 mgm.

Meningitis →
Irritable when moved – lethargic otherwise. Drowsy. Possibly convulsions.
C.S.F. cloudy – or purulent.
Cells 1000–10000.
Protein high. Organisms present.

Cerebral malaria →
High fever. Often convulsions.
Delirious – later semi-coma.
C.S.F. clear.
Cells up to 10, occasionally 20.
Blood film has malaria ++

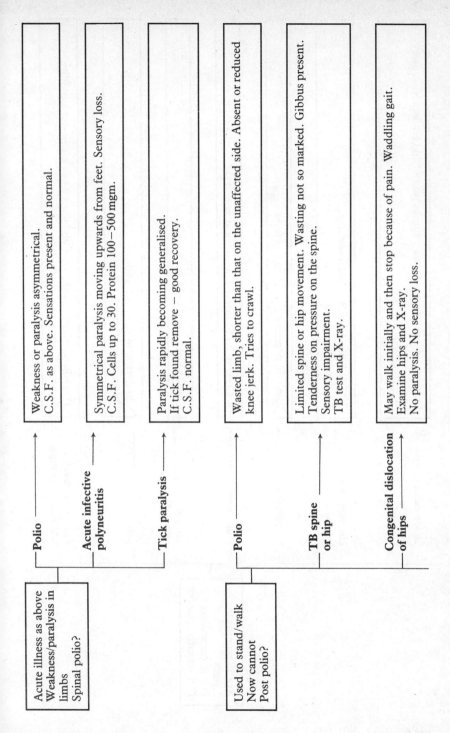

Acute illness as above
Weakness/paralysis in limbs
Spinal polio?

Polio → Weakness or paralysis asymmetrical. C.S.F. as above. Sensations present and normal.

Acute infective polyneuritis → Symmetrical paralysis moving upwards from feet. Sensory loss. C.S.F. Cells up to 30. Protein 100–500 mgm.

Tick paralysis → Paralysis rapidly becoming generalised. If tick found remove – good recovery. C.S.F. normal.

Used to stand/walk
Now cannot
Post polio?

Polio → Wasted limb, shorter than that on the unaffected side. Absent or reduced knee jerk. Tries to crawl.

TB spine or hip → Limited spine or hip movement. Wasting not so marked. Gibbus present. Tenderness on pressure on the spine. Sensory impairment. TB test and X-ray.

Congenital dislocation of hips → May walk initially and then stop because of pain. Waddling gait. Examine hips and X-ray. No paralysis. No sensory loss.

Age 18 months to 3 years
Has never walked
Polio in early infancy?

Sickle crisis → Examine for swelling/tenderness. Limbs painful and tender. No sensory loss. Check blood.

Unsuspected fracture → Palpate limbs carefully. Local swelling. Tender area.

Osteomyelitis → Pain – tenderness – swelling? – fever.

Polio → Wasting of limbs marked, and absent knee jerks.

Mental retardation → Check milestones. Limbs not wasted.

Cerebral palsy → Child hypertonic – not weak. Often has facial grimace also.

Severe bilateral dislocation of hips → Test whether knees can be fully abducted when knees and hips fully flexed – X-ray.

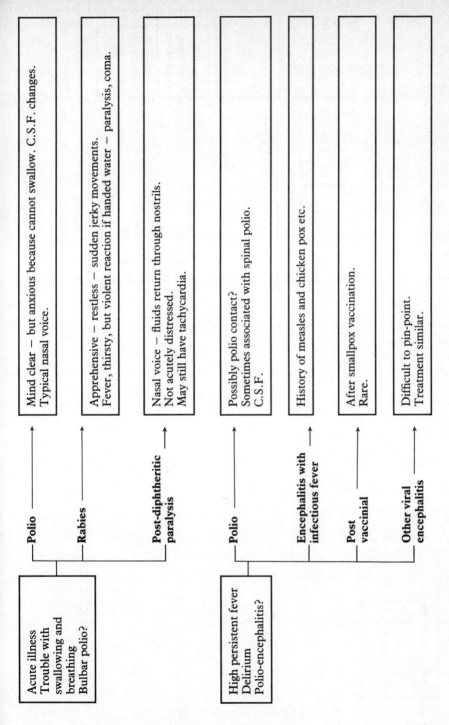

Acute illness
Trouble with
swallowing and
breathing
Bulbar polio?

Polio → Mind clear – but anxious because cannot swallow. C.S.F. changes. Typical nasal voice.

Rabies → Apprehensive – restless – sudden jerky movements. Fever, thirsty, but violent reaction if handed water – paralysis, coma.

Post-diphtheritic paralysis → Nasal voice – fluids return through nostrils. Not acutely distressed. May still have tachycardia.

High persistent fever
Delirium
Polio-encephalitis?

Polio → Possibly polio contact? Sometimes associated with spinal polio. C.S.F.

Encephalitis with infectious fever → History of measles and chicken pox etc.

Post vaccinial → After smallpox vaccination. Rare.

Other viral encephalitis → Difficult to pin-point. Treatment similar.

159

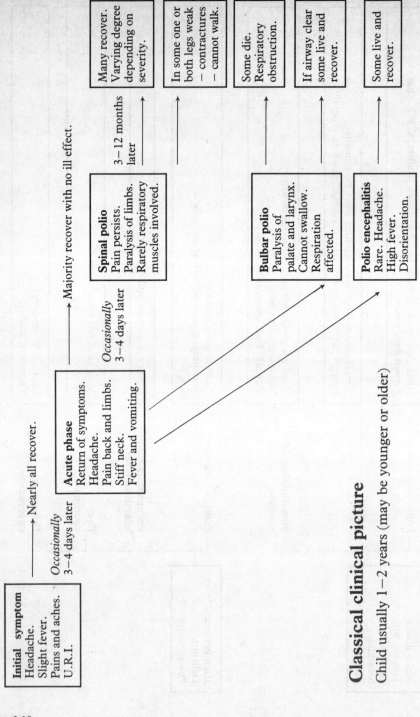

Initial symptom
Headache.
Slight fever.
Pains and aches.
U.R.I.

→ Nearly all recover.

Occasionally
3–4 days later

Acute phase
Return of symptoms.
Headache.
Pain back and limbs.
Stiff neck.
Fever and vomiting.

→ Majority recover with no ill effect.

Occasionally
3–4 days later

Spinal polio
Pain persists.
Paralysis of limbs.
Rarely respiratory
muscles involved.

3–12 months
later

Many recover.
Varying degree
depending on
severity.

In some one or
both legs weak
– contractures
– cannot walk.

Bulbar polio
Paralysis of
palate and larynx.
Cannot swallow.
Respiration
affected.

Some die.
Respiratory
obstruction.

If airway clear
some live and
recover.

Polio encephalitis
Rare. Headache.
High fever.
Disorientation.

Some live and
recover.

Classical clinical picture

Child usually 1–2 years (may be younger or older)

Treatment of poliomyelitis

After the acute phase there is some recovery of power in the muscle groups, of greater or lesser degree depending on the initial severity. This return of power is relatively rapid during the first 3–4 months and may continue up to 1 year. Because of this, the treatment is subdivided as that for:
● acute phase;
● home instructions and early follow up;
● further follow up;
● treatment of neglected cases with contractures.

Acute phase

Main aims at this stage are to:
– make the child as comfortable as possible;
– win the family's confidence and convince them that *something* can be done;
– teach the mother how to prevent contractures.

Note   In the peripheral hospital there are usually no mechanical respirators to treat respiratory paralysis and treatment of such cases will not be discussed.

● Admit to an isolation cubicle for 7 days, or until the 8th day of illness. Simple precautions – washing of hands, isolation of feeding utensils, cleanliness of attendants and correct disposal of linen and excreta are indicated.
● Establish a relationship with the mother.
● Cot of adequate size with boards under mattress and foot boards. Small pillows available for limbs. When in pain allow to lie in position of choice.

If unable to turn, see that child is turned over 2 hourly. When pain less, let the child lie with feet against foot board and small pillow under knees. The paralysed arms need support.
Or make the child lie prone with small pillow under ankles.
● Treat pain with analgesics – e.g. aspirin. Give regular dose so that the child is not neglected at night. Reduce in a few days when pain less. Hot moist towels or hot water bottles are of great help.

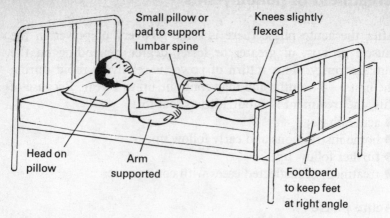

Small pillow or pad to support lumbar spine

Knees slightly flexed

Head on pillow

Arm supported

Footboard to keep feet at right angle

Nursing acute poliomyelitis

● No injections – they predispose to weakness in limb injected.
● Usual nursing care.
– Adequate fluid intake and nourishing diet.
– Check that the child is passing urine – feel for bladder daily – if palpable, apply gentle pressure and urine may pass. Try to avoid catheterisation. Recheck 4 hourly – if catheterisation necessary over some days, give antibiotic cover.
– Constipation common. Give suppository if necessary.
– Check respiration, pulse and swallowing reflex 4 hourly.
– If difficulty in swallowing, make the child lie on the side so that the secretions will not obstruct airway. Suction as necessary, to clear airway.
● Discuss with the mother the importance of the *position*, that if left alone, the child may have deformities. Carrying child on the hips will not be good, the knees should not be kept widely separated.

Do not carry on the hip

– If *sitting*, have a chair with a straight back with support for the arms and feet. Made to *fit* the child.
– If *lying*, it is an advantage to lie *prone* so hips are not flexed.

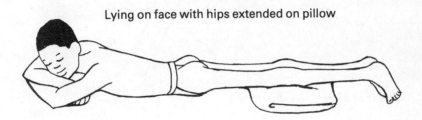

Lying on face with hips extended on pillow

Prevention of deformities

● Teach her how to stretch muscles gently, when pain and tenderness have gone.
● **Instructions for patients and relatives.**
● If someone is available to assess muscle power and chart – this can be a base line to observe future improvement.
  Muscle charting summarised.
  0 = No power.
  1 = Flicker of movement only.
  2 = Movement with gravity eliminated.
  3 = Movement against gravity.
  4 = Movement against gravity + resistance.
  5 = Normal power e.g. quadriceps.

Home instructions and early follow up

● Discuss the present care needed at home and teach the father as well as the mother how to do the exercises. Their attitude may be fatalistic, the child is 'finished' if she can no longer stand or walk – no further interest may be taken in her (or him). Show that you and all the staff in the ward do not think so.
– This child *can* be helped to walk again.
– This sickness *is* preventable.
– They should know this in case they have further children.
● Re-stress importance of position, the best position to sit and lie.

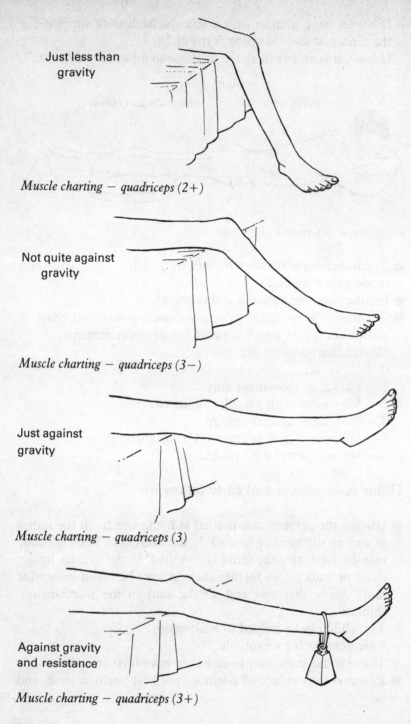

Just less than
gravity

Muscle charting — quadriceps (2+)

Not quite against
gravity

Muscle charting — quadriceps (3−)

Just against
gravity

Muscle charting — quadriceps (3)

Against gravity
and resistance

Muscle charting — quadriceps (3+)

- If the child is fit enough and there is a stream nearby, suggest they take the child and support him in the water. He may be able to do movements in the water that he cannot do on land.
- Appointment in 2−3 weeks. Take careful note of exactly how to find their house in case they do not attend.

Further follow up

If orthopaedic services or physiotherapist's advice available, then use them, even if it means sending the child some distance.

The book 'Poliomyelitis' by R.L. Huckstep (Churchill Livingstone 1975) shows what may be done, and is invaluable. Only a few points are mentioned here. If the child is more than 14 months old, **the main aim is weight bearing and walking**. Here are some of the things you can do.

Dropped foot only
- The shoemaker can fix a spring to the toe of the sandal connecting to a band below the knee.

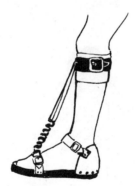

Spring for drop foot

Unable to bear weight due to quadriceps weakness
i.e. unable to bear weight on knee.
- Stablise by Plaster of Paris (P.O.P.) back slab − extending from the upper thigh to just above ankle.
- Easier to apply if child is prone.
- Remove back slab for drying for 24 hours.
- Return to child and apply crepe bandage.

165

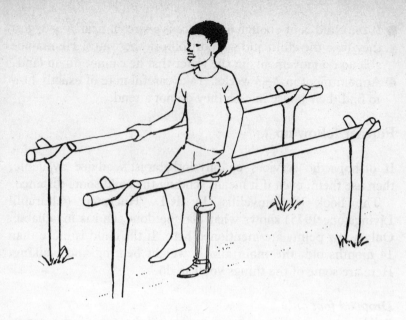

Parallel bars

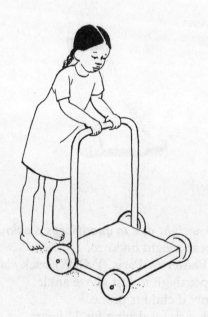

The walker

166

- To be worn in the day when practising standing and walking.
- Give extra support by making home-made parallel bars or a special walker.
- Change the P.O.P. back slab every three weeks – for 2 or 3 times.
- Some children have gained enough strength to manage alone. If not, and the mother is *co-operative*, speak with the family about sending the child to the nearest centre where expert advice can be given and calipers and crutches fitted and supplied.

Severe back weakness, as well as weak hips and legs

- This is difficult to treat and really needs an orthopaedic opinion and a physiotherapist.
- The following points are important.
- Posture – see that the child lies straight – and is turned regularly from side, to prone, to side and back.
- Sitting – should be on a special chair with back and side supports and foot rest, *made to fit* the child.
- Exercises – *in water* would help to make the most of any muscle power remaining.

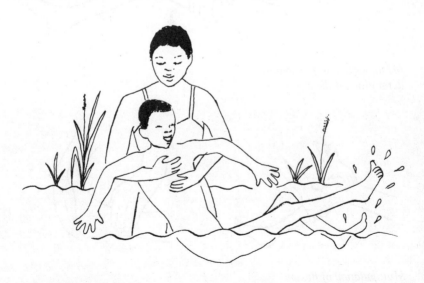

Exercising in water

A **spinal support** made from one of the new plastic materials may *prevent* a severe scoliosis and enable child to walk with calipers and crutches. Some will need a **wheelchair**.

Treatment of contractures in post-polio

- Causes are:
- imbalance of muscle groups;
- effect of bad posture in bed or on floor;
- bearing weight on a weak leg.
- Prevention is by stretching muscles several times a day, by parents at home.

Commonest contractures
- Hip – flexion with abduction.
- Knee – flexion with some posterior displacement.
- Ankle – tight tendo-achilles.

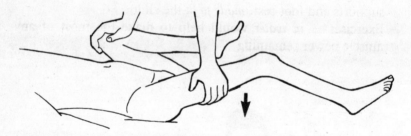

Manipulation of flexion/abduction deformities of the hip

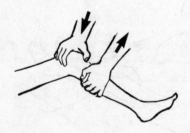

Manipulation of flexion deformity of the knee

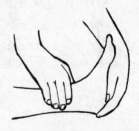

Manipulation of contracture of the ankle

168

Ideally those who have gained experience in specialised centres should treat. But possibilities are:
● mild contractures − active stretching;
● moderate − serial plaster casts;
● more severe − surgery with release of tight bands, etc.

Long term physiotherapy always essential and individuals may need calipers, wheelchairs and other equipment.

Who is to organise and do this treatment

The above outline of treatment has not been written down because it is thought that the nurse or an inexperienced over-worked doctor in the peripheral hospital can do it − but it was outlined to show what *could be done*.

Huckstep believes that a central teaching hospital in a country should be the hub of all the polio care.
● Peripheral doctor, physiotherapists, orthopaedic assistants, caliper makers, social workers are trained there.
● The more difficult cases are assessed and treated there.
● After training, doctors and other members of the team return to their areas and set up smaller units − for assessment, caliper making, to organise clinics and carry out straight-forward and operative treatment.

Only when the Teaching Hospital teaches a *team* able to re-produce the work in remote areas can children be prevented from becoming permanent cripples.

Prevention of poliomyelitis

The only effective way is by well planned community mass campaigns at regular intervals. This will require a high level of organisation.
● To give adequate notice to all concerned.
● To aim to get the under-4 year olds and particularly the infants.
● To get them to come 3 times.
● To have the vaccine adequately refrigerated during transport, storage and distribution.

169

Vaccine

- As strains are varied — best to use 3 doses of trivalent vaccine at intervals of 4 weeks, 3 drops each time.
- Minimum age, 1 month. Usually start at 6 weeks.
- Store at 2–8°C (not in freezing part of fridge).
- Transport in cold insulated boxes. Protect from direct sunlight.
- Booster doses at 5 years and 10 years.

If poliomyelitis is highly prevalent at a given time
- Injections of any sort are inadvisable in those with suspicious symptoms.
- However, if the child has to have an urgent operation, give injection of gamma globulin 1.5 ml/5 kg.

Looking back on aims

- **Prevent.**
- **Respect** those who have it, and give best care you can.
- **Make the community aware**
  - that you *can* prevent;
  - that you can get the crippled walking or mobile.

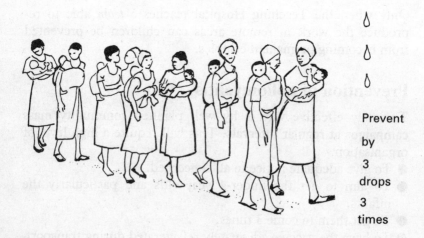

Prevent
by
3
drops
3
times

Aim to prevent

170

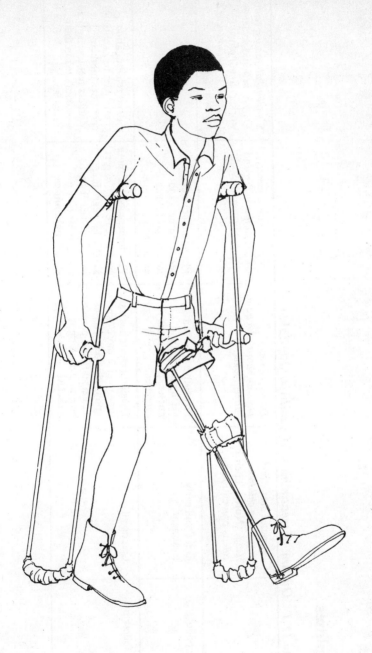

Aim to get the crippled walking

Facilities

Table 11.1 Outline of treatment with facilities available

	Interested doctor and nurses in a children's ward. (**Note** Their best role is prevention.)	Doctor, nurses, physiotherapist who trains caliper maker.	Physiotherapist, nurses, doctor, caliper maker and orthopaedic surgeon.	Simple rehabilitation centre. Staff as in 3 and social worker. Small physio. facilities. Workshop near a school and hospital.
Acute polio	Can do all early treatment.	Physiotherapist can teach mother (and nurses) posture and exercises.	Physiotherapist can teach mother (and nurses) posture and exercises.	
Early follow up	Can do all.	Physiotherapist has more time to give more expert knowledge re exercises. Teach staff and parents how to stretch tight muscles.	Physiotherapist has more time to give more expert knowledge regarding exercises. Teach staff and parents how to stretch tight muscles.	Attend rehabilitation centre. Get to know staff and other mothers. Mothers feel less isolated – encouraged in their follow up.

Further follow up	(Problem is lack of time.) Foot drop – could advise shoemaker to make toe spring. Can make P.O.P. back slabs. Could have parallel bars made on the verandah as pattern for the family. Could have a 'walker' to show design. Could have crutches made.	Physiotherapist more experienced in assessment. Give periods of intensive physiotherapy and teach mothers. Could take a man trained in simple leather work and teach how to make calipers and correct fitting of calipers. Learn how to mould spinal support. Do muscle charting. Help patients to walk and teach parents home follow up care.	Interested orthopaedic surgeon would have background knowledge of value in assessing and treating more seriously involved. Could train orthopaedic assistants. (Huckstep)	*Staff* geared particularly to rehabilitation. Time is not *snatched* from the acutely ill. Room for everything; for seeing patients, for the equipment, for the application of P.O.P. workshop for making calipers. A store for crutches and calipers. Periods in hospital could be relatively short if follow up at R.C. The community would be aware of problem and push for prevention.
Post polios with contractures	Could start exercises. Teach mothers best posture and exercises. Do serial P.O.P. and wedge. Know available referral centres and refer if necessary.	Personally supervise posture, exercises, and teaching mother. Do P.O.P.s and wedge. Arrange calipers, crutches, walkers.	Surgeon could assess initially. Operate to release contractures, and other procedures.	Follow up after operation could be done at R.C. Training centre for orthopaedic assistants, and caliper makers. Some children could attend nearby school.

CHAPTER 12

Anaemia

Anaemia is widespread. After protein-calorie malnutrition it is the second most common nutritional disorder in developing countries.

Anaemia presents clinically in 3 ways.
● The hundreds seen with moderate anaemia — pale and listless.
● The gasping, pallid child who comes to clinic in heart failure.
● The child presenting with some other illness with anaemia as a secondary and additional problem.

Is this necessary? What can be done?

Etiology

Five common causes
● Malaria.
● Infection.
● Hookworm and other parasitic infestations.
● Dietary iron deficiency.
● Sickle cell anaemia and other haemoglobinopathies.

The less common
● Haemorrhage.
● Folate deficiency.

Less common still
● Haemolysis due to G_6PD deficiency.

Certain causes are more common at certain ages.

Neonates
- Blood loss at birth (abruptio or 2nd twin).
- Bleeding from circumcision site or oozing umbilical stump.
- Haemorrhagic disease.
- Less common G_6PD deficiency.
- Blood group incompatibility.
- Poor maternal stores of iron.

Small infants
- Anaemia of prematurity.
- Infection.
- Poor iron stores due to maternal anaemia.

5 months – 1 year
- Malaria.
- Infections.
- Sickle cell anaemia.

One year onwards
- Malaria.
- Infection.
- Iron deficiency.
- Hookworm.
- Sickle cell anaemia.

and

less common
- Folate deficiency.
- Chronic or recurrent illness.

Understanding is also needed as to **how** the anaemia is caused.

Infection
- Particularly if very severe or prolonged, depresses the *formation* of red cells in the bone marrow.

Sickle cell anaemia
- There is *break down* (haemolysis) of red cells – iron is not lost – the spleen may be packed with iron. The child can be

175

anaemic yet overloaded with iron. Also, more commonly, anaemia is caused by sequestration of the erythrocytes in the spleen.

Iron deficiency

● Maternal iron deficiency leads to poor iron stores in the foetus and the newborn. The demands of growth in infancy lead to rapid utilisation of whatever body stores may be available. Infection with malaria in early infancy can precipitate severe iron deficiency anaemia with congestive cardiac failure.

Folate deficiency

● Necessary in the *formation* of red cells, may be deficient due to:
- poor intake – in malnourished child;
- haemolysis as in sickle cell disease;
- a greater need for it as in prolonged infection or malaria – or in pregnancy.

G_6PD deficiency

● An *enzyme deficiency* in certain children resulting in *haemolysis* and jaundice after taking certain drugs, e.g. aspirin, phenacitin, sulfonamides, primaquine and Vitamin K.

The hundreds of children with moderate anaemia. How can it be tackled in the clinic?

Know the normal values

Table 12.1

Age	Hgb		P.C.V.
	g	%	%
Birth	19	130	55
6 months–2 yrs	11	75	35
2–10 yrs	13	90	40
Adult	14.5	100	44

Note   PCV = Hgb × 3

Aim to find the cause (before commencing treatment)

History

Age   *Significant*

Neonate   Ask for history suggestive of multiple pregnancy; antepartum haemorrhage; preterm birth; circumcision or oozing umbilical stump; recent jaundice; infection; maternal anaemia with poor iron store.

Infants   Inquire about diet; recent high fever or infection.

Older   Inquire about diet; medicines; abdominal pain; infection; recent uvulectomy.

Family   Ask about history suggestive of sickle cell anaemia; any previous deaths amongst sibs.

Examination
Pulse Temperature Appearance Nutritional status Oedema Shortness of breath Pallor Jaundice Conjunctiva Spleen and liver enlargement

Tests
Initial
- Haemoglobin or P.C.V.
- Sickle cell screening test.
- Thick and thin smears for malaria parasites; presence of target cells, reticulocytes or nucleated red blood cells; lobes of neutrophils; hypochromia and anisocytosis.
- W.B.C. (if question of infection).
- Stool – hookworm?

In the majority of children you will have found the cause and commenced treatment by now.

If still in doubt, or if Hgb less than 7 g or P.C.V. less than 20

Table 12.2

On blood film	Suggests
● Red cells	
– small and pale;	Iron deficiency – infection – sickle cell anaemia.
– large;	
– normal.	Folate deficiency e.g. in kwashiorkor.
● Normoblasts (young red cells) present.	Bleeding.
	Rapid red cell formation e.g. sickle cell anaemia or haemolysis.
● Sickle cells.	
	Sickle cell disease. Do electrophoresis if possible.
● Haemoglobin electrophoresis.	Haemoglobin type.

Further tests – available in larger laboratories if diagnosis doubtful

● Reticulocyte count – if high as 8–10% suggests haemolysis.
● G_6PD enzyme.
● Bone marrow.
● Serum iron, folate and B_{12} estimations if possible.

If laboratory facilities not easily available

● Rule out common causes of anaemia (like malaria and hookworm).
● If in doubt *treat* with iron ⟶ There may be a response; check by noting reticulocyte count and Hgb.

● If no response, but has been prescribed iron. Take steps to make sure ⟶ *the patient is taking the medicine.* Very common cause of no response.

● If no response check the *dose* is sufficient. ⟶ Good response with adequate dose means *iron deficiency* was the probable cause of anaemia.

● If no response – poor absorption of iron? Therefore give by injection. ⟶ Response means *malabsorption.*

● If no response – not *utilising* the iron? Search for hidden infection. ⟶ May find *infection*, e.g. urinary tract, or nephritis, TB or other.

● If no source of infection found or if still no response ⟶ send blood away for further tests as mentioned above.

Remember
● It is possible to find sickle cell anaemia (S.S.) + hookworm in the same child or S.S. and iron deficiency.
● If you give iron to a person who is already overloaded, damage to internal organs like the liver, heart and pancreas can occur.
● For intramuscular administration of iron – calculate required total dose by weight, and Hgb deficit by the following formula: Total iron requirement (in mg) = Wt. in kg $\times$ (14 − Hgb in g/100 ml)
1 ml of Imferon provides 50 mg of iron.
Give in divided doses – and *stop.*
Recheck haemoglobin in 3 weeks.

- Always chart progress on a haemoglobin chart. Use weight chart for the purpose.
- When treating iron deficiency with oral iron, continue medication for 6 months *after* the haemoglobin is normal in order to replenish tissue stores.

Treatment of anaemia

Table 12.3

Type	Prevention by	Treat

Neonates
1 Blood loss
  ● Abruptio placenta
  ● Placenta praevia
	Antenatal and obstetric care.	If severe − marked pallor;
		      − persistent fast heart rate.
		− **transfuse**
		If less severe
		− **observe** $\frac{1}{4}$ hourly apex beat rate;
		− start course of intramuscular iron.
		Note Haemoglobin *not* a true indication of blood loss until after 24−48 hours.

● Bleeding from cord stump ● Gastrointestinal bleeding − 'haemorrhagic disease'	Clamp; rubber band safer than ligature. Vitamin K 0.5 mgm to immature.	Reclamp − and treat as above. Vitamin K 1 mg and treat as above.
● Bleeding circumcision wound	Arrange clinic facilities for circumcision.	Stop the bleeding. Suture. If anaemia is severe − transfuse. Moderate − A course of iron therapy. Give A.T.S. and penicillin if the circumcision was performed at home by a traditional practitioner.

2 Anaemia due to haemolysis
  ● ABO/Rh incompatibility
  ● G$_6$PD
	See neonatal jaundice.	

180

Table 12.3 (*contd.*)

Type	Prevention by	Treat
Immature babies and twins 6–8 weeks old with iron deficiency	Ferrous sulphate (60 mgm/5 ml) 30 mgm twice daily from age 2 weeks – orally.	● Imferon – Total dose (in mg) = Wt. (kg) × (14 – Hgb in g/100 ml). 1 ml Imferon = 50 mg of iron. Daily single dose of 0.5 ml. ● Continue with oral iron. ● Rarely need transfusion.
Infection	● *Check* for infection when anaemia not responding to iron. ● Leucocyte count. ● May be 'hidden' e.g. pyelitis, TB, osteomyelitis or salmonellosis.	● Treat specific infection. ● Good diet. ● If iron or folate deficiency present, treat. ● If no response, and anaemia is serious, or longstanding infection – transfuse. For moderate anaemia give blood 20 ml/kg. For severe anaemia give 10 ml/kg packed cells and repeat.
Malaria	Antimalarials from 3 months to 5 years. Teach mothers to treat attacks of malaria.	● Chloroquine and prophylaxis. ● Follow up charting Hgb on weight chart. ● Folate if anaemia severe or prolonged. ● Transfusion required sometimes.
Dietary iron deficiency	Start solids or egg at 6 months. Green leaf and liver at 8–9 months. Then good mixed diet.	● Moderate – Ferrous sulphate. 30 mgm/kg/day (Fe. sulph. paed. 60 mgm/5 ml). – Commence with Imferon if you wish. ● Severe. – Hgb below 45% or P.C.V. 15% + clinical picture. – Transfuse as above. ● Discuss diet.

Table 12.3 (*contd.*)

Type	Prevention by	Treat
Due to hookworm	Avoid exposure of skin by means of footwear.	● As for iron deficiency. ● Bephenium in a single dose of 2.5 g *or* Pyrantal 10 mg/kg to a maximum of 1 g *or* Thiabendazol 25 mg twice daily for 2 days *or* Levamisole 1 tab. for 1–4 yrs old, 2 tabs. for 5–15 yrs old.
Sickle cell disease	Prevention of crises ● Talk to parents about the disease. ● Attend S.S. clinic. ● Daily folate – weekly antimalarial chemoprophylaxis. ● Prompt treatment of infections. ● Immunisations. ● Avoid exposure to damp and cold e.g. staying in wet clothes. ● Carry card stating 'I have S.S.' and show at clinics and hospitals.	*Crisis* ● Analgesics for pain *as long as necessary*. ● Treat any infection/malaria. ● Maintain good hydration, by I.V. fluids if necessary. ● P.C.V. or Hgb daily. If Hgb below 4 g transfuse. ● Folic acid ● In skeletal lesions, danger of gram negative infections. If suspect– ampicillin or chloramphenicol

Type	Prevention by	Treat
Folate deficiency	● Prevent by adequate daily intake of green vegetables, liver, milk. ● Mixed feeding at 5–6 months. ● Malarial prophylaxis. ● Daily folate in S.S. disease.	Folic acid 2.5–5 mgm/day ($\frac{1}{2}$–1 tablet). If severe: injection 15 mgm I.M. Improve diet.
Chronic illness e.g. Rheumatoid – Nephritis	Treat streptococcal infection.	Treat condition. Transfuse when necessary.
Trauma Accidents/Burns	Accident prevention.	Remember *large* blood loss with fractures. Be ready to transfuse.

Summary of prevention

Normal child
● Mixed diet starting 5–6 months.
● Malaria prophylaxis $\frac{4}{12}$–5 years.
● Prevention and treatment of hookworm infestation.
● Prevent infections by immunisations, good hygiene, clean water, using latrines, etc.

Child with sickle cell anaemia
● Parents' awareness – S.S. talk.
● Sickle cell clinic.
● Chemoprophylaxis for malaria.
● Folate daily.
● Early treatment of infections.
● Prevent exposure to damp and cold.

Above plus

Treatment
● Consider treatment for those with P.C.V. below 30%.
● Must treat those below 20%.
● It is urgent – an emergency – to treat below 15%.

The treatment of the emergency

Child with severe anaemia and cardiac failure

● Take blood for all tests − not only haemoglobin, grouping and cross-match. Will need WBC and differential.
Infection?   Leukaemia?
Sickle cell screening test and haemoglobin electrophoresis.
May need sample for reticulocytes − blood culture, etc.
If facilities available − bone marrow.
● Diuretic (frusemide) ⎫ immediately.
  Digitalise   ⎬
● Hourly apex beat − chart.
● Cross match blood and give *packed* cells 10 ml/kg.
Delay often means death.
● Keep I.V. going with slow drip dextrose in ⅕th saline (if you had trouble getting into the vein) and repeat transfusion in 12−24 hours.

Blood transfusions

When considering whether transfusion is indicated or not, take the following into account.
● Haemoglobin and packed cell volume provide a good guide − but *not* the only one. Consider the patient's general condition.
● Laboratory facilities in a small hospital may not be reliable and there is a greater possibility of the danger of mismatched transfusion.
● Weigh up dangers of transfusion with dangers of *not* transfusing.
● **Before taking blood from donor, remember**
− Minimum haemoglobin should be 10 g/100 ml (70%).
− V.D.R.L. should be negative. Spirochaetes die in 72 hours in fridge and examination of a blood smear is not enough.
− Malaria is transmissible by transfusion.
− Icteric index − if serum is jaundiced, discard the blood.
− The patient can have a reaction on account of filaria antigen.
● **Collecting blood from donors**
− Use A.C.D. solution.

184

− Bottles should be autoclaved (not boiled).
− Careful grouping and cross-matching should be carried out.

Cross match Time: 1 hour usual and essential, but 15 mins. for emergency. In such a case the doctor takes the responsibility.

Storage of blood 14 days in the tropics. The temperature of the fridge must be 4−10°C. If more than 10°C, the blood should not be used.

Note on haemoglobin method
● Wait 15 min. before reading.
● EEL colorimeter. Choose an apparatus which allows you to standardise.
● Lovibond discs for haemoglobin estimation are available.
● Haematocrit.

CHAPTER 13

Respiratory Distress

Table 13.1   Notes on respiratory distress in children (excluding newborns)

Clinically	Possible cause	Treatment
Rapid breathing. Indrawing of intercostals. Flaring of the alae nasi. Usually fever.	**Pneumonia**	● **Antibiotics** 5–6 days. ● **Position** Do not sit a small infant almost upright in bed. The abdominal contents press upwards, and reduce lung expansion. If you wish, elevate the *head end* of the *bed*, and turn the child from side to side.

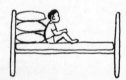

Poor position in bed

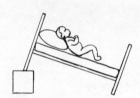

Good position in bed

| | | ● **Suction** as necessary.
 ● **Nasogastric tube feed** if necessary.
 ● **Oxygen** if cyanosed – but oxygen is rarely available in small hospitals.
 ● **If in cardiac failure** digitalise and give diuretic.
 ● 4 hourly **temperature chart**. |

Table 13.1 (contd.)

Clinically	Possible cause	Treatment
Pneumonia which is *not* improving, or else improved and relapsed.	**Empyema** Percuss both sides of the chest. If one side is quite dull — this may be fluid or pus.	● Call for more skilled help if available. ● After the usual history and physical examination, do **pleural tap**.

Position of pleural tap

		− Carefully position the child. The tap is made just below the angle of the scapula on the *dull* side. ● **If pus found, continuous drainage of empyema** is necessary.

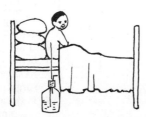

Drainage of empyema

		Tube from the chest is connected to a bottle with an underwater seal. ● **Give antibiotics** (after culture, if facilities available).

Table 13.1 (*contd.*)

Clinically	Possible cause	Treatment
In children under 2 years – cough with dyspnoea, struggling for breath, expiratory difficulty, chest looks 'blown up' or emphysematous, cyanosis, restlessness. Very fast heart rate. Patient febrile and toxic.	**Bronchiolitis**	● **Provide humidity** from a **steam kettle**. Sheets around 3 sides of bed. ● **Antibiotics** Broad spectrum – e.g. ampicillin. ● **Promethazine** 0.5 mg/kg 6 hourly if very restless. ● **Fluids** Usually too ill to suck. Either feed by nasogastric tube and remove each time, *or*, give I.V. fluids ($\frac{1}{5}$ saline in 5% dextrose) for a few hours. ● **If early cardiac failure** Digoxin. ● For those with **poor peripheral circulation**, consider hydrocortisone.
Persistent cough – often following measles or pertussis; – foul smelling sputum; – losing weight; – fever on and off.	**Lung abscess**	● X-ray (P.A. and lateral) to confirm and identify the position of the abscess. Send sputum for culture and sensitivity. ● Commence treatment with ampicillin plus cloxacillin given parenterally. Dose: 62.5 mg in children 0–2 years old. 125 mg in 2–10 years old × every 4 to 6 hours. ● If not longstanding, some get better with conservative treatment. But many need surgery. ● Postural drainage – and clapping for 10 minutes 3 times a day. (See notes on postural drainage.) Ask the child to cough when he is upright again. Delay postural drainage if child very ill.

188

CHAPTER 14

Two Genito-urinary Problems

Urinary infections

● This is the 'hidden' infection.
● It may present as:
− undiagnosed fever (P.U.O.);
− vomiting;
− failure to gain weight and loss of weight;
− lassitude;
− abdominal pain;
− frequency, urgency and pain on passing urine.
● It is important to make the correct diagnosis and treat, because a lower urinary tract infection, when untreated, passes up to the renal pelvis and can cause pyelonephritis with scarring of the kidney.
● If it occurs more than once in the same child, congenital obstruction should be excluded by doing intravenous pyelogram and micturating cystourethrogram. It is recommended that boys of any age and all girls under the age of 5 should be investigated. If such facilities are not available in your hospital, refer the child to a larger centre.

Diagnosis

Urine
● Mid-stream specimen.
− Protein increased − a trace or 1+ in non-catheter specimen is not necessarily pathological.
− Pus cells − if more than 10 per high power field, do gram stain, and check the organism.
− Culture done to:
  1 confirm organism if in doubt;
  2 check antibiotic sensitivity.

- Suprapubic aspiration.
- *Any* organism signifies urinary tract infection.
- Catheterisation should be avoided, if at all possible, because of the likelihood of introducing infection.

Treatment

- Most urinary infections are due to *E. coli* and respond to sulfadimidine or co-trimoxazole. Continue treatment for 10−12 days.
- Re-check urine in 5−7 days. If normal, re-check again in 1−2 weeks.
- If on initial re-check there is no improvement, culture the urine and give appropriate antibiotic.
- If there is a second urinary infection or a prolonged infection not responding to antibiotics − do I.V.P. to exclude malformations.

Oliguria and anuria − renal failure

Usually occurs in
- Acute and chronic glomerulonephritis. Exclude infected scabies as a cause.
- Shock following severe trauma, burns or dehydration (pre-renal failure). Early diagnosis will avoid parenchymatous damage.
- Accidental poisoning or poisoning by certain indigenous herbal potions.
- Transfusion reactions.
- Blackwater fever.
- Obstructive uropathy (post-renal failure).

Clinically there is vomiting, drowsiness, mental confusion and in some patients hypertension.

Treatment

- Treat cause if possible.
- In severe trauma or burns − give plasma or blood.
- In severe dehydration − I.V. fluids.
- If due to drugs − discontinue the offending drug.
- If transfusion reaction, give sodium bicarbonate to alkalinise the urine.

- In Blackwater fever, stop quinine – give chloroquine cautiously, and transfuse if patient is anaemic (haemoglobin <5–6 g/dl).
● Fluid intake must be restricted to avoid fluid overload. Amount has to be decided individually, depending on thirst, age and daily losses through sweating, temperature, vomiting and diarrhoae. Approximate amount is + 300 – 500 ml daily.

The nutritional intake should be 100 cal/kg/day to minimise catabolism using $\frac{1}{2}$–1 g/kg high class protein to keep a positive nitrogen balance. Nomograms for calculating body surface area are available. The formula used is:

Surface area (m^2) = weight $(kg)^{0.5378}$ × height $(cm)^{0.3964}$ × 0.024265. A rule of thumb method for estimating body surface area by weight alone is:

$$\text{Surface area } (m^2) = \frac{4W + 7}{W + 90}$$

$$W = \text{weight in kg}$$

Avoid fruit juices, especially orange juice which contains potassium.

● Check progress by means of the following procedures.
– Daily intake and output chart.
– Daily weight – increase warns of fluid retention.
– Daily B.P.
– Electrolytes – potassium – most vital – death may follow a high blood level.
– Sodium bicarbonate and blood urea.
● Food – by nasogastric tube if necessary.
● If anaemia (haemoglobin <5–6 g/100 ml) give transfusion of packed red blood cells.
● If hypertension is present and cannot be controlled by fluid restriction, give hypotensive drugs, e.g. hydralazine and/or propranolol.
● Mannitol 0.5–1 g/kg of 25% sol. over 10–20 minutes (maximum 25 g), or frusemide 1 mg/kg I.V. over 30 minutes, has been advised in pre-renal failure.

Response is indicated by increase of output, and then – diuresis. This may take up to a month to occur – so encourage parents not to give up hope even though response is slow.

CHAPTER 15

Meningitis (Acute Purulent)

It is extremely important to be good at 'spotting' this condition *early* before there is permanent brain damage or death.

Important facts

Acute purulent meningitis
● *It is more common* in the *very* young — in some instances up to 80% are below 2 years.
● Clinically it presents *differently* in neonates, so they will be dealt with separately.
● Clinical presentation is often *like* acute malaria with fever and convulsions — **so always check for and exclude meningitis**.

Suspect if a child diagnosed as having malaria is treated and *still* has fever, with or without convulsions.
● If a child is treated for a convulsion and has been put on 8 or 12 hourly sedation but *still* has convulsions.
● If a child diagnosed as having pneumonia with fast breathing and cough, who is receiving antibiotics, starts convulsions or is not getting better.
● If any child looks *more sick* than she did 2 days ago, in spite of treatment.

Whenever in doubt, do a lumbar puncture.
● *The 3 commonest organisms are*:
− H. influenzae;
− Meningococcus;
− Pneumococcus;
but in 50−60% of patients *no* organisms are found in the C.S.F. (possibly because of antibiotics given outside).

192

The following refers to 'purulent' meningitis *not* TB meningitis which has a slow and insidious onset.

Table 15.1

Infants	All	Older children
● Full or bulging anterior fontanelle.	Fever and restlessness. Irritability. 'Cries when lifted'. Lies on side. Vomiting.	'Headache'.
● Refusing to feed.	Stiff neck (except neonates).	
● May be vomiting.	Delirious. Convulsions.	
● Fast apex beat.	Semi-coma. Coma.	

Examination
- ● Note especially increased heart rate and temperature.
- ● Note if mind is not clear — may be drowsy, or hyperactive, or delirious.
- ● Remember to check the infant's anterior fontanelle (it is often forgotten when the hair is thick).
- ● Train yourself to recognise *'increased resistance'* of the neck — even before it is really *'stiff'*. If present, a lumbar puncture must be done.
- ● **Learn the 'head-lag test'**
- — The child must not be crying. If the child *is* crying you cannot do the test satisfactorily. The child must be lying on his back — you gently take hold of both upper arms, in the way adults do when they are going to lift a child to the sitting position. Do it slowly and hold the child's arms for a moment before you begin to raise up the child.
- — The normal response is for the child to flex the neck *first* before allowing himself to be lifted forward.
- — In meningitis, it hurts to lift the neck forward so the child lets it fall back at first. (Head lag 1.)

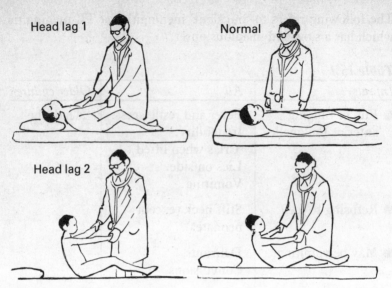

Meningitis — the head lag test

– Finally when he *is* sitting up he brings the neck forward. (Head lag 2.)
– This is called a positive 'Head lag' test.
– Children with meningitis have it. Those with malaria do not.

If the test is positive, a lumbar puncture must be done.

Diagnosis

Confirmed by lumbar puncture.

C.S.F.
● Appearance — If cloudy or purulent, even if no laboratory facilities — *treat* as meningitis.
● Before sending to the laboratory, keep a small quantity to examine yourself.
● **Examination**
– Do gram stain.
– Carry out a leucocyte count and differential.
● **Typically**
– C.S.F. Leucocyte count — hundreds to thousands.
– Gram Stain — Gram positive pneumococcus.
    or

194

Gram negative e.g. H. influenzae and meningococcus.
- Protein — Normally 20–40 mgm. Raised in meningitis.
- Sugar — Normally $\frac{2}{3}$ of blood sugar i.e. about 50–70 mgm.
  Reduced in meningitis — usually below 40 mg.

Blood
Leucocyte count raised and mainly polymorphs. Hgb and haematocrit drop quite rapidly. Malaria parasites may or may not be present.

Outcome in meningitis

● If no antibiotic . . . . Death
● If antibiotic given but:
- too late;
- dose too small;
- stopped too soon;
- did not reach meninges;
- organism insensitive.
The smaller the infant

⎫ Subdural collections of fluid
causing pressure on brain
or
adhesions causing hydrocephalus
and neurological damage
or
brain damaged child. ⎭

● If early diagnosis and
  antibiotic administered:
- in high dosage;
- for sufficient time;
- intravenously for 4–5 days.
If organism unknown use a
combination of antibiotics or
a very broad spectrum one.

⎫ Good result.
Normal child. ⎭

Treatment

Antibiotic

● Classically **triple therapy**.
- **Penicillin** to cover meningococcus and pneumococcus.
- **Chloramphenicol** to cover H. influenzae.
- **Sulfadiazine** also for meningococcus (but many strains resistant to sulfa and penicillin now).
● Drugs given intravenously into I.V. tubing.

195

- Dosage high for first few days.
- Drugs given in rotation 2 hourly.

Dose

- Benzylpenicillin 10−20 mg/kg daily. Give 6 hourly I.V. 2.5 mg/kg at 6−12−18−24 hours.
- Chloramphenicol 50−100 mgm/kg daily, divided into 4 doses and given 6 hourly I.V. 2 hours later e.g. 2−8−14−20 hours.
- Sulfadiazine 75 mgm/kg 6 hourly I.V. at 4−10−16−22 hours. After 4 days reassess and hope to reduce chloramphenicol.
- Alternatively ampicillin 100 mgm/kg/24 hours.
  Divide by 4 and give 6 hourly I.V.
  Results as good as triple therapy.

Note   If the intravenous needle blocks in the night, give antibiotics I.M. and restart I.V. in the morning, **but do not miss a dose**.

Fluids

- An intravenous drip should be put up for the first 4 days at least so as to give I.V. antibiotics. But watch daily intake and beware of over-hydration.
- Pass a nasogastric tube for feeding if the child is very ill and drowsy.
- Allow the child to drink as soon as he is willing.

Sedation

Often necessary for a few days because of convulsions.

Vitamin B

Indicated because of antibiotics.

General

- Routine care same as for semi-comatose patient. Hence special nursing care needed.

- Nurses observe general condition hourly – and vital signs 4 hourly.
- 4 hourly temperature chart essential – it indicates *progress*. Continue this until temperature below 100°F (37.8°C) for 2–3 days and general condition improved.
- Routine check for anaemia – malaria, and treat if necessary.
- Do tuberculin test.

Day by day follow up in hospital

- Check 4 hourly temperature graph – temperature should be below 100°F (37.8°C) (on *4 hourly chart*) for 7 days before antibiotics can be stopped.
- Check general appearance and alertness e.g. doing any new things like calling parents, holding head up, wanting to eat?
- Check intake and output and state of hydration – any vomiting. Often occurs at first, but should not restart.
- If infant, check anterior fontanelle – getting tense? Measure head circumference daily.

Danger signals

- Temperature over 100°F (37.8°C) after 4–5 days of treatment *or* fresh rise in temperature after it has come down.
- Vomiting or twitching after 4–5 days of treatment.
- Infant's head enlarging.
- Sunset sign.

These all suggest
either – subdural collection of fluid,
or – adhesions blocking free flow of C.S.F.
A subdural tap or referral for more skilled care are necessary.

When no danger signals

- Temperature falls gradually, child's mentality improves, and he starts talking, drinking and eating.

- If child is malnourished, and has even *moderate* anaemia, a blood transfusion helps to boost up the general condition.
- If on *triple therapy* — *organism unknown*
- Reduce chloramphenicol to usual dose 50 mgm/kg/day on 4th–5th day and stop it on 7th–9th days.
- Reduce sulfa drug to usual dose also 4th–5th day and stop altogether 7th day.
- Continue penicillin till temperature below 100°F (37.8°C) on *4 hourly chart*.
- If on *ampicillin*
- Reduce dose to 50 mgm/kg/24 hours by 5th day and stop when temperature below 100°F (37.8°C) for 7 days.
- If in doubt, repeat lumbar puncture.
  If cells below 60, antibiotics can be stopped.

Meningitis in neonates

- Think of it when *any* neonate is sick.
- Think of it also in the most efficiently run maternity units.
- Think of it especially after infected deliveries, but even after a 'normal' delivery.
- Think of it when a newborn on the third day onwards:
- 'just doesn't look well';
- 'doesn't want to suck';
- 'sucks a little and vomits a little';
- 'seems to have gone pale';
- 'the eyes seem to be turning upwards or to one side';
- 'the temperature is up a little';
- 'the temperature is down a little';
- 'the anterior fontanelle feels big';
- 'the baby stopped breathing for a moment'.
- **In other words**, everything is very vague, **except for a persistently fast apex beat**.
- **It is no good expecting a stiff neck** — you don't get one.
- You don't even always get a bulging fontanelle. Of course you will *eventually* but by then it's rather late. Try to diagnose *before* the bulging fontanelle.
- Also you cannot do the head lag test — because the head lags normally.
- When in doubt, do a lumbar puncture.

Organisms

The commonest are *E. coli*, staphylococcus and streptococcus.

Treatment

- Essential to give antibiotics by intravenous route.
- Move child to the place where those most experienced in looking after I.V. fluids are.
- Send C.S.F. specimen to the laboratory for the usual tests.
- *Antibiotics* depend on what is available but avoid chloramphenicol and sulfa drugs.
  Give either:
- benzylpenicillin 30 mg/kg daily with gentamicin 3 mg/kg every 12 hours by intramuscular injection or slow intravenous infusion;
- if gentamicin is not available, ampiclox 75 mgm 6 hourly I.V. initially then I.M. and oral
- ampicillin 100 mg/kg/day divided into 4 and given I.V. (reduce dose in 4 days);
  or
- if neither of these newer antibiotics available, then as a last resort give benzylpenicillin as above and streptomycin 5 mgm/kg/day I.M.

Subdural collection of fluid or subdural abscess

Occurs over one or both parietal lobes.

How? a membrane forms round a collection of purulent C.S.F.

Result Antibiotic cannot reach the fluid inside the membrane. C.S.F. is drawn *into* it by osmosis through the membrane and so it *enlarges* and causes increased intracranial pressure. The head and the anterior fontanelle enlarge. Vomiting and twitching may occur. **It will not go away on its own.**

Treatment

Subdural tap
When danger signals occur e.g. generalised convulsions during convalescence, vomiting; focal convulsions; hemiparesis or neurological abnormalities; bulging fontanelle; impairment of consciousness or an unsatisfactory clinical course; a subdural tap should be attempted through the lateral angle of the anterior fontanelle.

Aspirate both sides. The child may have to be transferred to a larger centre where skilled care is available.

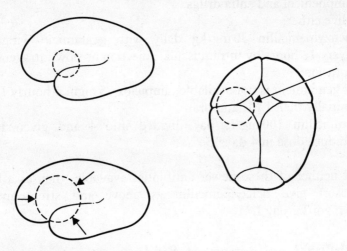

Subdural collection of fluid

Procedure
Check anterior fontanelle *is* open. Shave anterior to a line drawn from ear to ear.

Procedure
● Sterile procedure.
● Infant held with vault of head towards operator.
● Skin cleansed well. Sterile towel applied.
● Using lumbar puncture needle, the lateral angle of the anterior fontanelle is punctured gently.

- The needle then penetrates the dura, the stylet is removed, and if there is fluid it is caught in a test tube.

$\frac{1}{2}$–1 ml of clear C.S.F. is normal.

In subdural collection the fluid is yellow, turbid and comes easily.

Result
- If no fluid obtained on one side, the other side may be tried.
- If fluid is present not more than 30 ml/day should be removed.
- If diagnosed early and tapped daily, the condition may resolve.
- If no improvement after 2–3 weeks, surgical removal of the sac is necessary.

CHAPTER 16

Some Common Skin Conditions

Rash — cause unknown

Ask mother

● What soap does she use to wash the child and the clothes? Some children have a reaction to detergents.
● What does she add to bath water? Some mothers add powerful disinfectants that are irritant.
● Is she applying menthol, Dettol, or any home remedy to the skin?
● Can she get water easily, or does she have to carry it a long way? If in rural area, is there a stream nearby? Is the child washed daily?
● Is the child on any medicaments?

When possible cause found — discuss with the mother e.g. if irritant, stop using it. Apply calamine lotion.

Scabies

● Always itching — worse at night.
● Often secondarily infected and so scabies is masked.
● In children usually generalised, in adults localised to specific areas.
● If child has it, the mother and other members of the family also have it, so look at their hands and arms.

Treat
If secondary infection present, treat first and only then treat underlying scabies.
   Treatment of scabies — benzyl benzoate for all the household.

- Day 1
- Wash child all over with soap and hot water.
- Dry quickly with clean towel.
- Apply benzyl benzoate *all over except* the face — both where the rash is seen and where it is not seen.
- Dry in the air.
- Wash and boil all clothes.
- Day 2
- Ordinary wash with soap and water.
- Day 3
- Have clean clothes and bedding ready.
  Repeat first three procedures from day 1.

Repeat again in 4 days until cured. If not improving, check if *all* the people in the household took treatment.

Pyoderma

Skin infection — pustules — abscesses — impetigo
- Cleanliness vital.
- Hexachlorophene soap useful.
- Antibiotic creams often cause skin sensitisation and are best avoided.
- Try mercurochrome in water. Bacitracin ointment useful in impetigo.
- If severe and especially in newborns give penicillin systematically.

Furuncles — boils

- Aspirin if pain (or other analgesic if available).
- Procaine penicillin if severe or extensive.
- Incise *as soon as* fluctuant.

Ringworm

Scalp
- Shave hair and burn.
- Whitfields ointment for some weeks.
- Griseofulvin may be used for widespread or intractable infection. Dose 10 mg/kg daily in 2−3 divided doses.

Body
- Whitfields ointment b.d. Commence $\frac{1}{2}$ strength. Continue for 10 days after skin clear.
- If severe griseofulvin for 2–3 weeks.

Feet
If acute with blisters:
- soak in warm potassium permanganate 1:8000;
- when acute phase subsided – Whitfields ointment $\frac{1}{2}$ strength b.d.

Fungal infection of skin folds (Moniliasis intertrigenous

- Nystatin and steroid lotion or cream b.d.

Tinea versicolor

Yellow areas of skin varying from the size of a pin head up to several inches. May be on trunk, neck or face.
- Responds to Whitfields ointment. Not to griseofulvin.

Otitis externa

- Paint with 1% gentian violet in water. If severe apply polymixin with hydrocortisone.

Papular urticaria

Itchy papules that child scratches.
- Look for mites e.g. in wooden bed or cot. Apply D.D.T. to patient and bed.
- Calamine lotion.
- Oral antihistamine while itching troublesome.

Creeping eruption

Due to skin invasion of larvae.
- Treat – thiobenzadole 25 mgm/kg b.d. for 5 days orally.

Infantile eczema

Itchy rash, sometimes weeping, on face and in flexures in young children.

● Calamine lotion with 3% crude coal tar.
● Keep as cool as possible.
● Avoid soap to areas of rash. Clean with oil.
● Sedation if necessary at night.
● Severe exacerbations may need hydrocortisone cream for a few days only. If steroid continued longer there may be a severe relapse when steroid finally stopped. Avoid other more powerful steroidal preparations except for hydrocortisone.
　　When discontinuing it, do gradually over 2−3 days.

● CHAPTER 17

Problems in Diagnosis

Diagnostic puzzles are not such great problems if the possibilities are considered, and the ways to investigate for these possibilities are known. Here are a few common problems.
● Large abdomen, and mass in the abdomen.
● Failure to thrive.
● Undiagnosed fever.
● Behavioural and emotional problems.

Large abdomen

Table 17.1

Consider	Notes and tests
Commonest cause Malnutrition	The 'pot belly'. Often associated with heavy load of ascaris. Weight chart.
Generalised distension but no obvious fluid or palpable masses ● Megacolon	History of constipation. If rectal examination shows a full rectum consider fecal impaction. Treat with laxatives and enema. If rectum is empty consider Hirschsprung's Disease.
● Peritonitis	Looks ill. Later there is obvious fluid.
● Septicaemia with paralytic ileus	Especially in neonates. May have infected umbilicus and jaundice also.

206

Table 17.1 (*contd.*)

Consider	Notes and tests
● Meconium ileus in the newborn	
● Typhoid fever	Slow pulse. Low white blood count. Widal +.
● Intestinal obstruction for any cause	Vomiting persistent.
● Atresia — bands in newborns	Upright abdominal X-ray shows fluid levels.
● Volvulus — intussusception	
● Following trauma: Injury to spleen or liver Penetrating injury to gut	May have internal bleeding, but not enough to tap. Close observation. Be ready to do laparotomy. Peritonitis developing.
Ascites present	
● Congestive cardiac failure	Oedema elsewhere. Weak rapid pulse.
● Glomerulo-nephritis	Facial oedema. Raised B.P. Do urinalysis.
● Nephrotic syndrome	Oedema marked — albuminuria. ++
● Hepatic cirrhosis	Onset gradual. In late stages oedema on the feet. Urine — normal. No breathlessness.
● Tuberculous peritonitis	Not an acute onset. Positive Heaf test. High E.S.R. Responds to antituberculous drugs.
● Constrictive pericarditis or pericardial effusion (e.g. endomyocardial fibrosis)	Pulse poor volume. Raised jugular venous pressure.
● If no obvious cause, do diagnostic tap: — with strict sterile precautions;	

Table 17.1 (*contd.*)

Consider	Notes and tests
– after emptying the bladder; – in midline between umbilicus and pubis. Then you can: – examine fluid; – find enlarged spleen, liver or mass by abdominal palpation.	
Spleen and/or liver enlarged ● Sickle cell disease	Sickle testing. Genotype.
● Thalassaemia	In areas where it occurs.
● Tropical splenomegaly	Many respond to daily antimalarials given for a long time.
● Malaria	Recurrent infections in highly endemic areas.
● Amoebiasis and amoebic liver abscess	Amoebae *not* usually found in stool at this stage. If abscess – liver tap and drain (closed method).
● Pyogenic liver abscess	From umbilical infection or blood-borne.
● Salmonellosis	Looks ill – fever – loose stools.
● Septicaemia	Especially in neonates.
● Tuberculosis	When miliary, especially in small children.
● Hydatic cyst Schistosomiasis Kala-azar	In areas where these conditions occur.
● Infectious hepatitis ● Cirrhosis of liver	Possibly no jaundice. Do liver function tests. Basic cause often not found; may be hepatitis, malaria, pyogenic infection of umbilical vein, following neonatal jaundice, or malnutrition.

Consider	Notes and tests
In the infant	
● Septicaemia	
● Haemolytic disease	
– Infectious mononucleosis	Blood film.
– Leukaemia and Hodgkins	Blood film. Bone marrow. Biopsy.
– Tumours: Burkitts	Responds within days to cyclophosphamide.
Hepatoma	Laparotomy.
Neuroblastoma	
– Rare storage diseases	

Palpable mass	
Lower abdominal mass	
● Bladder	

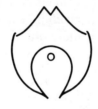

Distended bladder

Consider	Notes and tests
– Stricture or urethral valve	
– Neurological imbalance	As in coma – poliomyelitis. Sedated child especially if on I.V. fluids. Meningomyelocoele.
● Haemotocolpos	In the 11 – 15 year old girl who has never menstruated.
● Pregnancy	
Renal causes	
● Congenital abnormalities	Confirmed at laparotomy, especially if I.V.P. not available.

Table 17.1 (contd.)

Consider	Notes and tests
– Horse shoe kidney – Polycystic kidney or kidneys	

Congenital abnormality of the kidney

Consider	Notes and tests
● Hydronephrosis *Other discrete masses* ● Faecal ● Ascaris balls	Check blood and urine. I.V.P. if available. Send for specialist care. Enemas. Danger of obstruction if piperazine given in usual doses – give less and more often.

Ascaris masses

Consider	Notes and tests
● Mesenteric adenitis TB or other ● Deep abscesses *Tumours* ● Ovarian ● Dermoid ● Burkitts	Heaf test. Responds to anti-tuberculous treatment if TB. White count up. Fever. Laparotomy.

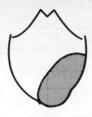

Ovarian tumour

Consider	Notes and tests
● Neuroblastoma ● Wilms ● Others	

First steps in investigating failure to thrive

Table 17.2

Birth to five months

Cause	Due to	To do
Poor sucking reflex	Prematurity. Small-for-dates. Cerebral palsy or brain damage. Hare lip. Congenital heart disease. Debility due to: anaemia; infection.	History of pregnancy. Weight. History of labour. Examine baby. Apex beat. Check liver. Haemoglobin. Do urinalysis. Blood count and culture if facilities available.

Table 17.2 (contd.)

Cause	Due to	To do
Insufficient breast milk	Maternal cause. Twins.	Examine mother — breast; — general. Alternate breast feed with milk by cup.
Premature babies tube fed in hospital	E.B.M. given but mother's milk decreases. Sometimes *quantity* made up with *glucose water* and so milk is *too dilute.*	Add prepared artificial milk to E.B.M. Baby to breast *as soon as possible.*
Artificial feeding	Too dilute. Too infrequent. Giving diluted cereal preparation (or other food) and no milk.	Question mother in detail. Discuss ways to give milk.
Emotional deprivation	Orphan. Maternal separation.	Family history. Find mother substitute.
Anaemia	Prematurity.	Haemoglobin. Prevent with oral iron. Treat with Imferon.
Hidden infection	Pyelitis. Osteomyelitis.	Do — urinalysis; — X-ray. Appropriate antibiotic.

Five months onwards

Cause	Due to	To do
Inadequate calorie intake		
● Stopping breast feeding too early.	Bottle appears to be a good substitute. Ignorance of value of breast feeding.	Create community awareness. Use breast feeding counsellors. Treat feeding bottles as **killers**.
● Bottle feeding.	Too dilute — too infrequent.	
● Starting mixed feeding with low energy density foods.	Ignorance.	Education — from school onwards.
● Starchy diet.	Ignorance. Father gets solids (meat). Child gets liquid soup and porridge. Poverty.	Discuss with mother. Make use of nutrition rehabilitation centres. Take social history.
Poor appetite		
● Infections.	Malaria. G.I. infection — feeding bottles.	Chemoprophylaxis. No bottles in hospital. No advertisements. No nurse to bottle feed.
	Measles. Pertussis. TB Respiratory infections.	Immunise. Immunise. Vaccinate. Health education re fresh air in houses. Avoidance of smoke.
● Anaemia.	Malaria — Hookworm. Sickle cell.	Blood smear. Stool examination. Sickle cell test.

Table 17.2 (*contd.*)

Cause	Due to	To do
Increased metabolism Chronic infection.	Tuberculosis. Pyelitis, Osteomyelitis etc. Hidden abscesses.	Heaf − Chest X-ray. Urinalysis. White blood count. Blood culture.
Malignancy.	Leukaemia − Tumours.	Complete blood count.
Failure to absorb and assimilate	Repeated purges and enemas.	History. Instruct.
	Intestinal parasites e.g. Giardia.	Stool test.
	Post diarrhoea lactose intolerance.	Stool for reducing substance. Stop milk temporarily.

Summary of approach in failure to thrive

Diagnosis in the individual child

- ● History of pregnancy
- − labour;
- − birth weight;
- − feeding: maternal separation?
- − family: twins? a broken family? − social and economic situation.
- ● Recurrent diarrhoea?
- ● Weigh and chart on Road to Health Chart.
- ● Examine
- − General and systemic examination.
- − Infant sucking well?

- Examine mother's breasts for retracted nipples – milk secretion.
- Test weigh.
● Possible tests
- Haemoglobin.
- W.B.C.

If anaemia is found carry out serum iron and folic acid estimations.
- Heaf.
- Urinalysis.
- Blood: Malaria? Sickle cell?
- Stool: – for ova or – for lactose.

Check the stools for the presence of mucus or blood, and for excess fat.
Chest X-ray if Heaf negative and TB suspected.
X-ray bones if osteomyelitis?

Prevention

● National consciousness
- Value breast feeding – up to 12–18 months.
- Feeding bottles are **killers**.
- Mixed feeding from 5 months. Use edible oils and fats.
- How to feed infants and children.
- No home treatments including purges or enemas.
● Weight card for every child an essential aid in growth monitoring.
● Chart weight. Give immunisations – vaccinations – chemoprophylaxis against malaria.
● Health education – nutrition education.

Sustained or intermittent fever more than 2 weeks in young child

No obvious clinical signs, except anaemia and possibly enlarged spleen. Adequate antimalarials already given. Conditions marked XX are those most common, and X those common in one area. You may wish to mark your own.

215

Table 17.3

Consider	Notes and tests
Infections	
Hidden abscesses	
● Retropharyngeal ('cold' abscess)	TB? Do Heaf test.
● Lung	Sputum. X-ray chest.
X ● Empyema	Re-examine chest, remembering percussion. Pleural tap if dull.
● Appendix abscess	
X ● Deep abdominal	
● Deep inguinal	
X ● Liver	Re-check liver size. Possibly liver tap.
● Pelvic	Rectal examination.
● Subphrenic	Radiological screening.
● Perinephric	Local tenderness.
● Pott's	Tender over spine or on compressing spine with short press on head. X-ray.
● Pus in one of the large joints	If the patient is a carrier of the sickle cell gene then most likely causative organism is a salmonella.
Other infections	
X ● Otitis media	Careful examination of the ear drum.
● Mastoiditis	Local tenderness.
● Pericarditis	Listless − tachycardia − increased cardiac dullness − possibly pericardial rub. X-ray.
● Bacterial endocarditis	Evening temperature. Cardiac murmur. Positive blood culture if no recent antibiotics.
XX ● Urinary tract infection and pyelonephritis	Urinalysis and culture − 2−3 times.
● Osteomyelitis	Deep palpation over bones. X-ray if tenderness.

Consider	Notes and tests

XX ● Tuberculosis
   – if miliary in
     infant?
	Tuberculin test. X-ray chest.
	Ziehl Neilson test on morning –
	gastric aspirate collected with sterile
	precautions.

– if bone or joint?	X-ray bone or joint.
● Relapsing fever	Temperature chart with few days fever and remissions of 1–2 weeks. Responds to penicillin, tetracycline or chloramphenicol.
● Visceral larva migrans	Increased w.b.c.s and eosinophils. Treat with thiabendazol.
● Meningitis	Usually obvious signs – but tuberculous meningitis may be of insidious onset. H. influenzae meningitis may present with fever as the most prominent symptom initially.
Bacteraemias	
X ● Salmonellosis	Blood culture – Widal.
● Shigellosis	Stool – microscopy – pus and blood – culture.
XX ● Septicaemia	More common in sickle cell disease – Gram negative frequently.
Virus infections	
X ● Hepatitis	Simple liver function tests. Bilirubin.
● Mononucleosis	Peripheral blood smear for abnormal mononuclear cells.
● Dengue	Low white cell count.
X ● Other viral infections	
X ● Amoebiasis	Stool examination.

Table 17.3 (contd.)

Consider	Notes and tests
Dehydration and high external temperature	Often in motherless babies with insufficient fluid intake. Overdressed babies.
● Heat stroke	In very hot weather.
XX Drug reaction	Hospitalised child on too many drugs. As fever persists, more drugs added.
Auto immune	
● Rheumatoid arthritis	Fever may be the only symptom for weeks.
Blood and malignancy	
X ● Sickle cell disease	Blood for sickling − genotype.
● Burkitt's lymphoma	Remember may occur anywhere in the body.
● Hodgkins	Chest X-ray may show hilar gland enlargement.
● Leukaemia	White blood count, differential. Bone marrow.
● Neuroblastoma	
X ● Other malignancies	Biopsy − laparotomy − other examinations.
Add others in your area	

P.U.O. check list

Table 17.4

Fever – For how long? Continuous? On and off? T° ranges from...to....	**Family** Anyone sick? Coughing? Jaundice? Diarrhoea? Died? Child living with mother? Motherless?
Other symptoms Pain?...Listlessness?	**Environment** Live in town? Village? Number sleeping in room? Water supply? Sewage disposal? Mosquitoes? Other?
Drugs or other treatments?	
Past history Discharging ear? Diarrhoea? Sore throat? Vomiting? Appetite? Change in personality? Recent infectious fever?	

Table 17.4 (contd.)

T°	Enlarged lymph glands	Fundi ....
Pulse	Chest dullness	Ears ....
Respirations	Heart dullness increased	Throat ....
Weight	Murmur	Rectal ....
Looks ill	Abdomen deep palpation	
	Liver .... Spleen	

White blood count	X-ray – chest	**More specialised tests**
differential	– spine	Bone marrow.
Hb/P.C.V.	– long bones	A.S.O.T.
Blood culture.	– other	Radiological screening.
Sickle cell test.		Biopsy.
Bilirubin.	*Urine*	Monospot for infectious
Liver function test.	Mic. Culture	mononucleosis.
Widal and other agglutination		Widal test and other agglutination
tests e.g. proteus; brucellosis.	*Stool*	reactions.
Other culture.	Mic. Culture	
Tuberculin test – Heaf.		
E.S.R.		**Special tests for conditions in your**
Cerebrospinal fluid examination.		**area**

Behavioural and emotional problems

In any given year between 5 and 15% of children suffer from disorders of sufficient severity to handicap them in their everyday life. Deviations from normal are not uncommon but when they are severe and persistent and become socially handicapping, intervention is needed.

Examples of behavioural problems

Emotional disorders
● Change of personality – has become withdrawn and sad.
● Temper tantrums.
● Refusing to eat.
● Night terrors.
● Excessive fears.
● Inattention at school – teacher complains – punishment doesn't help.
● Not doing at all well at school as regards work.
● Not playing with other children.

Conduct disorders
● Wild and aggressive behaviour.
● Stealing in an otherwise normal child, whose family are not poor.
● Bullying and fighting.

Overactivity

Possible causes

● Present illness or state of malnutrition, e.g.
– kwashiorkor associated with a change in personality and poor appetite.
– primary tuberculosis associated with lethargy and poor performance at school.
● Previous brain damage either at birth or later, e.g. meningitis or cerebral malaria.

- ● **Mentally retarded child** as yet undiagnosed.
- − Down's Syndrome.
- − Microcephaly.
- − Other forms of mental retardation.
- ● None of the above, but **a feeling of undue anxiety or inner conflict in the child's life**. Particular symptoms do not follow particular causes.

  The symptoms depend on:
- − the child's age and development;
- − the past life history;
- − the particular family and home situation;
- − the relationships with mother, father, brothers and sisters and others;
- − perhaps a recent happening or factor of stress.

The *reasons* for the anxiety are not *thought out* by the child: he or she may have no awareness of the reasons for a certain behaviour. The following are some common reasons which are found.

- − **The feeling of not being loved** by one or both parents. This may be due to their attitude to the child, or following separation from the parents. The separation may, in the parents' eyes, be for a *good* reason, e.g. education. The young child does not think this way − all he or she knows is that she is put far away from the person she loves most, and needs most.
- − **The feeling of not being able to achieve the high academic standards** expected by the father. This has been known to result in hysterical paralysis especially at examination time.
- − In some areas, **the fear of charms, spells and evil spirits** and what they might do. These fears are handed down from the parents in the same way the fear of snakes or scorpions is handed down.

  Mother becomes sick, or grandfather dies, a trading venture fails, or the crop is spoilt; 'Someone has done this'. Shutters are tightly closed at night to keep out evil spirits. The child imbibes the sense of danger lurking in the dark ready to harm; evil spirits are whispered about who seek out a victim and cast an evil influence.

Why we should try and tackle these problems

They are time consuming and when one has many patients, it is much quicker and easier to treat pneumonia and malaria. But:
● the parents very often have been to many other sources of help, and received none;
● the symptom may be as distressing to the child and the family as other physical symptoms;
● this change in behaviour *may* be the only symptom of a physical disease;
● when it is *not* a symptom of physical disease, it will be a symptom of a probably more painful emotional disease. Even without psychiatric training, if we take time to understand, we can often help.

However *time* is important — so a special time of at least an hour has to be set aside.

Outline of plan

Decide if the child's behaviour is abnormal
● Age and sex appropriateness.
● Persistence.
● Life circumstance.
● Severity and frequency of symptoms.
● Socially handicapping.

Rule out physical causes
● Listen to complaint initially.
● Take a brief routine history.
● Do a thorough physical examination.
● In many children the cause will be either self-evident e.g. brain damage in a child who convulsed for 6 hours, or it may be highly suggestive, e.g. primary tuberculosis. In such a case, a further investigation — e.g. a Heaf test — will then be done.

Dealing with the others
History from parent
This is obtained usually from the parent who first came, but the ideal is to talk to both the parents.

- ● Complaint
- – Let the parents describe as much as they want to.
- – Ask their reaction to it and what happened then.
- – When did it start – is it continuous – did anything make it better or worse?
- – Any other complaint?
- – What do the parents think is the cause of the complaint?
- ● Development
- – Place in the family – Type of delivery – feeding – How long breast fed?
- – Any separation from mother?
- – Milestones –

Head up at.		Smiled at	. . . .
Sat up at		Stood up at	. . . .
Walked at		Fed himself at.	

- – Sleep – Goes to sleep easily? Wakes at night? Bad dreams?
- – Sleeps in the day?
- – Appetite good? Normal? Poor?
- ● Type of child
- – Personality – Happy – Anxious – Withdrawn – Hyper-active – Any special fears – Attitude to sex?
- ● Previous illness
- – Any handicaps? High fever for a long time?
- – Any convulsions or history of coma?
- – Any change in behaviour after an illness?
- – What treatment given? Traditional treatments. (These may be frightening, e.g. uvulectomy, scarification, branding etc.)
- ● Family
- – Father – Lives with family? If away, for how long? His work? What kind of person? Relationship with child?
- – Mother – Has been separated from child? Does she work? Relationship with child?
- – Other close members of the family.
- – Brothers and sisters – Discuss each in turn – What are they like? – Relationship with patient. From the *way* the mother answers you can tell what she feels about them.

  You will learn who are most valued in the family – Those who do well at school? The boys?
- – Grandparents – Influence on family strong?

224

- School
  - If child goes — Reaction to it — How is he getting on?
  - What do parents think of the school?
    Not strict enough?
  - Has child got playmates or friends?
  - Is child anxious about going to school?
    Is he punished?
- Now the mother has overcome her anxiety of the interview, ask her the *sensitive* questions.
  - What punishments has the child had for the complaints?
  - Sometimes the mother thinks the child has had a 'charm' or spell put on him or her, but she doesn't want to say this to hospital staff. If you think this is possible — ask her what she thinks of people who are said to put 'charms' on other people, and so give her an opening.
- Any recent change in the family's situation or the child's situation — e.g. one parent going abroad, or child being sent to live with grandmother.
- During this discussion observe the child.

Talk to child alone if older.
Does he/she know the reason for the consultation?
- Ask about the complaint — What happens — How it happens — Why?
- Don't press with questions if child does not want to talk.
- Ask about family: Father — What is he like?   What does he do?   Does he do things with you?   Or play with you?   And so on down the family.
  Home — What does he like doing best there?   With whom?
  School — What is it like?   What are the children in the class like?   Any special friend?   What are the teachers like?
  Sleep — Any fears?   Any fears of any sort?
  If old enough — ask if she could have 3 wishes, what would she wish for most?

Talk to teacher if this seems advisable.

Treatment

- Deal with *present illness* and explain to parents.

- If *brain damage* present, explain to parents how it happened. Also tell how it may be avoided with future children, as this will be their fear. Try to remove their sense of guilt — explain it is not their *fault*, and it is not due to anyone else wishing them harm. These things happen all over the world. But nowadays we know more and can often prevent these things.

   In a hyperactive brain-damaged child, sedation with phenobarbitone can help. Say you would like to see them again — from time to time. Your interest is also a help to the parents.

- If the child is **mentally retarded**, it is more difficult. There is often no specific cause that can be given to the parents. It is often a relief to them to hear the true facts, even though it is a shock. Many will accept this as one of the trials of life, without bitterness.

- **Dealing with anxiety**

- When the probable cause comes to light to both the doctors or nurse and the parents, the way to solve it may also become evident, e.g. if a 2 year old has been sent off to grandmother when the new baby arrived, it is not too difficult to bring the child back to the mother and father.

- When highly intelligent parents wish their son to shine scholastically, and he fails, they may be brought to understand that he needs their love not for what he achieves but for himself alone.

- Fears of evil spirits, spells and charms are more difficult to deal with, as in all probability the parents have the same fears.

226

CHAPTER 18

Emergency Treatments

When a child collapses or stops breathing

● Do not give nikethamide or other analeptics. They are dangerous.
● Do not give oxygen first.
● Do not leave the patient unattended and run for help.

Very often the air passages are blocked with mucus, feed or vomitus **so**

● If possible, suck out. If not, lift up the lower end of the body to allow fluids to drain out, until the airway is clear.
● Lie the patient flat and keep chin supported.
● Do mouth-to-mouth resuscitation – or use resuscitator if it is nearby.
● When breathing restarts give oxygen, if you have it.

If a child is pulseless and there is no heart beat

● Give a single short press on the front of the chest *or* do cardiac massage if you have been trained to give it to children and babies.

Hyperpyrexia

High temperature 104–105°F } Most commonly malaria
(40–40.6°C) } especially if no other signs
of infection or of early
measles.

Note **Aspirin is not the specific treatment for malaria.** It brings down the temperature.
It does not deal with the cause.

Chloroquine is the drug to treat malaria.
● **Injection** if very high fever or vomiting.
Dose depends on *weight* not *age*.
Dose − 5 mgm/kg (2½ mgm/lb)
e.g. 10 kg child − 10 × 5 = 50 mgm.
Read ampoule because strength varies − some 30 mgm/ml, some 40 mgm/ml and some 50 mgm/ml.
Parenteral chloroquine can cause cardiovascular collapse in young children and infants. Use only when absolutely necessary.

Pass a nasogastric tube and administer further doses of chloroquine through the tube.
● **Tablets** Chloroquine = 150 mgm base.

Table 18.1

	Up to 1 yr.	1−2	3−5	6−12	13−15
Initial	½	1	2	2	3
In 6 hours	½	¾	1	1	1−2
Day 2−5 (daily)	½	½	½	1	1−2

Aspirin 60 mgm/yr of age 3 times a day till temperature drops.

Sedation **To prevent convulsion** e.g. phenobarbitone.

Tepid sponge or put under fan.

Hourly temperature chart.

Emergency treatment of convulsions

(For neonates see under Neonate section)

Aims in the following order

● Stop convulsions and prevent further ones as well as prevent injury.

- Find cause.
- Treat cause.
- Follow up.

Stop convulsion

- Lie flat − remove pillow.
- Lie on side − so mucus drains from mouth.
- If on nasogastric drip − stop immediately.
- Sedate with *fast acting* drug.
- Paraldehyde 0.2 ml/kg (0.1 ml/lb) I.M.
  Follow up with slower but *longer acting* drug.
- Diazepam (Valium) 0.5 mgm/kg.
- **Do not** force a spatula between teeth *when convulsing*. When jaw relaxes insert spatula gently if possible.

Find out cause if not already known

Routine is always the same.

History
- When started?   Any other convulsion?
- Any other symptoms?   Home treatments?

Examination
- Temperature Pulse Respiration Skin normal? Signs of infection?
- Character of respirations?   Indrawing intercostals?
- Liver and spleen palpable?   Stiff neck?
- Mouth − pharyngitis, infection?   Koplik spots?

Lab. tests − if necessary
- Blood − malaria?   Leucocyte count; dextrostix.
- Urinalysis.
- C.S.F. examination.

Commoner causes

Malaria
- Convulsions vary from slight spasms to prolonged fits in

cerebral malaria. Neck usually supple but if increased resistance is felt, do lumbar puncture to exclude meningitis.
- Heart rate fast and respirations increased in proportion to heart rate.
- Spleen usually palpable.

Meningitis
- Child cries when lifted. Infants have bulging anterior fontanelle. Stiff neck in *older* infants and children. Often have an associated or preceding respiratory infection. Lumbar puncture confirms.

Early measles
- Before rash – Injected conjunctiva.
- Mouth – Koplik spots.

Upper respiratory infection
- Look at ears and throat.
- Adenovirus infection a common cause of febrile convulsions.

Pneumonia
- Respirations 60–120/min. Indrawing of intercostals. Flaring of nose. Signs in chest.

Any other severe infection
- Large abscesses; septicaemia; urinary infection.

Tetanus
- Spasms recur. Risus sardonicus. Unable to suck or swallow.

Treat cause

Follow up

- If fever
- – tepid sponge or fan *until temperature comes down.*
- – aspirin 60 mgm/year of age.
- Note time convulsions started. If continue for 10 minutes after sedation given, more sedation may be necessary.
- Maintain convulsion chart and hourly temperature chart.

230

- Sedation and possibly aspirin will be necessary 4–6 hourly for 2–3 days.
- Keep child where she can be *seen* by nursing staff – at all times.

Children with recurrent convulsions

With fever

- Spend time talking with parents about the necessity of preventing *malaria*.
- Therefore consider *chemoprophylaxis*.
- Order stock for parent to take home of **chloroquine** and **aspirin.** 6–10 tablets of each
- Explain to the mother the dose of each to give to the child if fever develops in the night. Also tell her to bring the child to the clinic the next day.

Recurrent convulsions, fits or spasms without fever

- Possibly epilepsy or brain damage.
- Send for skilled opinion if available.
  If no specific cause found – anticonvulsants may be ordered. To be continued for 2 years after the last seizure.
- – Phenytoin (Epanutin) and/or phenobarbitone.
- – Valproic acid (Epilim) and/or phenobarbitone.
- See child every week or two initially as the appropriate dose for each child must be found. If too little given, there will be recurrence. If too much, child will be drowsy, ataxic or show other side effects.
- If there is difficulty in controlling the seizures more expert advice should be sought.
- Remember every convulsion or fit has the potential of *brain damage*.

Emergency treatment of unconsciousness

Aims

- Ensure clear airway.

- Treat shock if present.
- Find cause and treat.

Ensure clear airway

- Lie on side.
- Suck out oro-pharynx using a mechanical sucker if available.
- Support chin or insert airway.

Treat shock

- Take pulse and B.P. If both low, start I.V. fluids.

Find cause

Know likely causes. The following have been found in order of frequency at one rural hospital.
- Cerebral malaria.
- Ingestion of poison
  - sometimes a local herbal potion;
  - sometimes tablets;
  - think of poisoning with berries e.g. Datura poisoning.
- Alcohol
  - may be taken in local potion;
  - may be taken 'for fun'.
- Post convulsive state
  - convulsions not seen by anyone.
- Hysteria
  - often a divided family;
  - examination time (if a school child).
- Meningitis
  - but usually there are preceding symptoms.
- Encephalitis
  - may be associated with infectious fever.
- Hyperpyrexia.

Less common
- Cerebral abscess
  - often associated with chronic discharging ear.
- Head injury
  - child injured some days previously — has subdural haemorrhage.

- Metabolic conditions affecting the C.N.S. e.g. Diabetes mellitus; uraemia; fluid-electrolyte imbalance; tetany
- rather rare. Do blood chemistries if facilities available.

- Vascular conditions like haemorrhage, thrombosis, embolism, subdural haematoma
- rare. A history of head injury may be present. Check B.P. and examine the cardio-vascular system.

In certain areas
There would be other known causes specific to the area.

History
- Recent symptoms − Trauma − Home remedies − Alcohol − Recent infectious fevers − Anyone else in family ill?

Examine
- Temperature − Pulse and respiration rate − Blood pressure − General appearance − Restless? − Smell on the breath? − Stiff neck, character of respirations, neck stiff or supple? − Signs of trauma? − Discharging ear?

Laboratory investigations
- Blood − malaria parasite;
  - leucocyte count;
  - sugar, urea, electrolytes, calcium.
- Urine − urinalysis;
  - sugar and acetone.
- C.S.F.

Table 18.2

Possibilities	To do
If − no localising neurological signs, or possibly slightly increased neck resistance (meningism); − no signs of trauma; − raised, normal or low temperature; **probably cerebral malaria.**	− start chloroquine 5 mg/kg I.M. − pass a nasogastric tube. − blood slide for thick drop exam. If positive for malaria give more chloroquine through nasogastric tube. − start I.V. fluids. − start B.P. chart.

Table 18.2 (contd.)

Possibilities	To do
If history of alcohol ingestion or typical smell from breath and no other signs **probably ingestion**.	– I.V. fluids fast. – suck out stomach contents through the nasogastric tube. – check B.P. every 15 mins.
If ingestion of poison (other than paraffin)	– I.V. fluids. – if child conscious, wash out stomach (unless more than 3 hours since ingestion). – if skilled help available to insert cuffed endotracheal tube, wash out while still unconscious.
If increased neck resistance or stiff neck – fever **probably meningitis/ encephalitis**.	– do lumbar puncture. – keep foot of bed elevated 24 hours. – examine C.S.F. and treat if positive.
If hyperpyrexia – delirium and malaria excluded **suggests encephalitis**.	– check on recent infectious fevers. – reduce temperature by sponging and fan. – if *any* doubt about malaria, treat. – careful lumbar puncture. – elevate foot of bed for 24 hours.

Possibilities	To do
If previous history of fits − although none observed this time **consider epilepsy.**	− arrange admission for full examination − epilepsy?
If − history suggestive − temperature − pulse − respiration normal − blood pressure normal − eyelids flicker − arm remains elevated when examiner lifts it up **consider hysteria.**	− admit child for further observation and discussion with relatives.

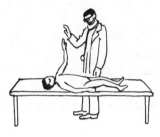

Diagnosing hysterical coma

If − high B.P. e.g. 180/120 **suggests hypertensive** **encephalopathy due to** **glomerulonephritis.**	− examine urine. − give antihypertensives e.g. mag. sulphate 50% 0.1 ml/kg−0.2 ml/kg/dose or hydralazine 0.3 mgm/kg/dose. Repeat in 6 hours if necessary.

Table 18.2 (contd.)

Possibilities	To do
If – none of above – urine sugar + + + + acetone + **probably diabetes.**	– do blood sugar and treat for diabetes.
If – no relative present to give history – and no diagnosis made from examination.	– send for recent contacts of child – enquire re trauma, missing tablets and alcohol.

Emergency treatment of severe anaemia

Child may have:
● extreme pallor;
● gross oedema;
● marked breathlessness;
● rapid, thready pulse.

This suggests **cardiac failure** in addition to anaemia.

Aims

● Prevent imminent death **but also vitally important – diagnose cause of anaemia so as to treat and prevent recurrence.**

Common errors

● Transfusion
– without treating cardiac failure;
– too much blood;
– too fast administration of blood.
● Transfuse correctly and then realise that blood samples were not taken for required tests – so no proper diagnosis.

236

Procedures

- Allow child to be in position of greatest comfort.
- Treat cardiac failure (if present).
- Diuretic — frusemide intramuscularly 0.5−1.5 mg/kg.
  Repeat in 4−8 hours.
  If improved give *orally* 1−3 mg/kg daily.
  If not give intramuscularly as at first.
- Digoxin 0.02−0.04 mg/kg/day.
  For rapid digitalisation half the oral dose may be given by injection.
  Check and measure the dose correctly.
- Take blood for all tests that may be required e.g. full blood count, sickle cell, malaria, group and X match. Keep some blood and reserve for more tests if required.
- Order blood transfusion — calculate amount for transfusion 4 ml packed cell or 6 ml whole blood/kg raises the haemoglobin by 1 g/dl. Give 5−10 ml/kg whole blood i.e. less than usual because of failing heart.
  Order enough blood to give second transfusion in 12−24 hours.
- Give packed cells, or sedimented cells if the blood bottle has been standing for some time.
- Routine history and physical examination.
- After diuretic is given and blood available and ordered, start setting up I.V. infusion so as to save time when blood arrives. Because of oedema it is often difficult to insert needle in the vein.
- If malaria is diagnosed avoid giving full dose (5 mg/kg) of chloroquine by injection before transfusion. Better to give half the dose — observe effect and give the other half in 1−2 hours when transfusion is in progress. Better still, give orally since absorption of chloroquine from the gut is rapid.
- Treat the cause of anaemia when diagnosed.

● CHAPTER 19

Hospital Diets

In all communities where malnutrition is prevalent, the feeding of sick children in hospital should receive special attention. This is because most of the children admitted to hospital for diseases other than malnutrition are suffering from various degrees of undernutrition. This gets worse during an acute illness for the following reasons.

● The accompanying anorexia reduces the food intake of the child.
● Because of the traditional customs and practices the child may have been put on a light diet, or starved, or given purges or enemas.
● All acute illnesses cause tissue breakdown and loss of nutrients from the body.

Dietary care of children in hospital is an important part of their therapeutic care.

This section is in 3 parts. Part 1 is intended for the relatively large hospitals with a paediatric ward. For such institutions a paediatric ward diet is described. Part 2 is intended for the smaller rural units with a handful of beds assigned for paediatric admissions. Because of the small number an individual approach is needed in the construction of a diet. Part 3 is intended for quick reference for dietary advice in cases with a deficiency of specific nutrients.

1 Routine Ward Diet

A specimen ward diet for a paediatric ward might be as follows:

6.00 a.m. – 1 slice (1 oz) bread spread with 2–4 g margarine or peanut butter.

6–7 fl ounces tea containing approximately 60% milk and sugar.

10.00 a.m. – 2 oz paw paw cut into small pieces and 5–6 ounces of porridge containing 43% fresh milk, 8% maize flour, 12% eggs and 2% sugar.

12.00 noon – 5–6 oz rice or stiff porridge.

3–4 oz mince meat containing 50% mince meat, 5% fish meal, 2% oil.

3 oz soup containing 7% carrot, 7% turnip, 15% spinach and bone broth.

3.00 p.m. – 1 slice (1 oz) bread and 2–4 g margarine.

6–7 fl oz tea as at 6.00 a.m. Half a fresh orange.

6.00 p.m. – 5–6 oz rice. 3–4 oz mince as at lunch, or beans, or groundnut stew, and 3 oz soup.

2 The Individual Menu-Counselling Parents

Feeding the child in hospital – from birth to five years

The baby from birth – 3 months

There is no medical indication for withholding breast milk. During an illness:

● **Breast feeding is a must. Bottle feeding is dangerous.**

● If the mother has to be out at work for 6 or 8 hours every day, **feed with cup and spoon not feeding bottles. Use modified low solute formula.**

Germs grow inside the teat and the inaccessible parts of the feeding bottle. Contaminated feeds cause loose stools and its associated dangers. Bottle feeding inside the hospital should be discouraged.

● The baby *doesn't need* cereal or anything else, at this age.

Remember

– **Breast feeding is essential.**

– **Feeding by bottle is risky and must be discouraged in the hospital.**

– **Cup and spoon are relatively safe.**

Table 19.1 Average intake of a child who is eating well

Food	(g)	Cals.	Prot. (g)	Fat (g)	CHO (g)	Ca (mg)	Fe (mg)	Vit. A (i.u.)	Thiamin (mg)	Ribofl. (mg)	Niac. (mg)	Vit. C (mg)
Bread	30	74	2.1	0.2	16.0	3.40	0.30	–	0.2	0.1	0.2	–
Margarine	2	15	–	1.7	–	0.08	–	56				–
Tea	212	119	4.5	2.1	20.0	159.00	0.13	91	0.055	0.198	0.17	2.3
Breakfast		208	6.6	4.0	36.0	162.5	0.43	147	0.26	0.3	0.37	2.3
Porridge with eggs	156	112	5.6	4.7	12.3	90.0	0.80	280	0.55	0.16	0.16	0.6
Paw paw	56	22	0.4		5.2	11.4	0.20	568	0.02	0.02	0.02	34.0
Sugar	10	40	–	–	10.0	–	–	–	–	–	–	–
Mid-morning		174	6.0	4.7	27.5	101.4	1.0	848	0.57	0.18	0.36	34.6
Rice	155	132	2.8	0.16	28.8	1.86	0.31		0.022	0.011	0.37	–
Mince	100	137	12.4	9.80	–	14.00	1.70		0.050	0.110	2.70	–
Soup	80	9	0.7	0.08	1.4	34.00	0.56	530	0.016	0.040	0.24	14
Stiff porridge	162	226	5.7	0.84	49.0	2.35	1.30		0.032	0.019	0.39	–
Mince	100	137	12.4	7.80	–	14.00	1.70		0.050	0.110	2.80	–
Soup	80	9	0.7	0.08	1.4	34.00	0.56	530	0.016	0.040	0.24	14
Lunch with rice		278	15.9	10.04	30.2	49.9	2.6	530	0.09	0.16	3.4	14

Food	(g)	Cals.	Prot. (g)	Fat (g)	CHO (g)	Ca (mg)	Fe (mg)	Vit. A (i.u.)	Thiamin (mg)	Riboff. (mg)	Niac. (mg)	Vit. C (mg)
Lunch with stiff porridge		372	18.8	10.72	50.4	50.4	3.6	530	0.10	0.17	3.4	14
Bread	32	80	2.2	0.2	17.1	3.60	0.35		0.019	0.013	0.22	0
Margarine	3	23	–	2.5	–	0.12	–	85	–	–	–	–
Tea	212	119	4.5	2.1	20.0	159.00	0.13	91	0.055	0.198	0.17	2.3
Orange (½)	70	37	0.6	–	9.1	21.00	35	21	0.060	0.020	0.14	31.0
Tea		259	7.3	4.8	46.2	183.7	0.83	197	0.13	0.23	0.5	33.3
Rice	110	94	2.0	0.11	20.4	1.3	0.22	–	0.015	0.008	0.26	–
Mince	113	155	14.0	11.10	–	15.8	1.92	–	0.057	0.124	3.16	–
Soup (no vegetables)	46	–	–	–	–	–	–	–	–	–	–	–
Supper		249	16.0	11.2	20.4	17.1	2.14	–	0.07	0.13	3.4	–
Average total daily		1215	53.3	35.1	170.4	514.8	7.5	1722	1.13	1.01	8.03	84.2
Recommended allowance 1–3 yrs.		1130	40			400	7	2000	0.6	1.0	6	35
3–6 yrs.		1510	50			400	8	2500	0.8	1.2	8	50

To keep the cup and spoon really clean enough for a baby, pour boiling water over them before feeding. After feeding, wash well and store in a covered container.

The baby at 4–6 months
● **Breast feeding is best**.
● If the mother has to work, then feed with cup and spoon because feeding bottles are dangerous and should be discouraged.
● **Fruit**   Now baby can take:
– orange juice;
– mashed paw paw;
– half mashed ripe banana.
● The next new food is the local cereal (often made from maize) in the form of gruel. But all such gruels have low content of energy and other nutrients. Hence add $\frac{1}{2}$–1 teaspoon of fat or edible oil to each cup.
● The baby takes a month or two to get used to this, his first real solid food. At about 5 months when he's used to it, **add body building foods to the cereal**, like:
– fresh milk;
– powdered milk (avoid condensed milk);
– ground crayfish or any small fish (start with a little);
– egg yolk;
– boiled and mashed groundnuts or beans.

Also at 5 months start **sieved vegetables** – green leaf (e.g. spinach), paw paw, egg plant and pumpkin.

Starting new foods
All babies suspect something new – they taste it, pull a face and spit it out.

The trick is to be patient and not to start a struggle. Just offer 2–3 teaspoons and wait till next feed. Try again. He'll spit it out again!

But suddenly after 3 or 4 days the baby may decide he likes it. Then he can't get enough!

Warning – **Only start one new food at a time.** Allow time for the baby to get used to one food before introducing another.

Once the baby knows what the new food feels and tastes like, add one of the body building foods like pounded groundnuts. Stick at that for 2–3 weeks before introducing another food to the baby.

The baby at 6–9 months
● **Breast feeding is still the best food for the baby.**
● If the baby is being offered milk, then feeding by cup and spoon is safe. Feeding bottle is not.
● Now the baby really needs *different* foods to grow *big* and *strong* and later on *clever*!
● Given below is a suggested menu.

Early morning breast feed

Breakfast
Cereal with milk powder;
or pounded crayfish;
or pounded groundnuts or beans;
or lightly boiled egg;
or the local bean preparation for children, i.e. skinned and pounded. Add to the above ¼ teaspoon of edible oil.
Fruit.

Lunch
Advise to choose one of these.
● Green vegetables mashed up with tomato, a little palm oil and stock from bone.

● Meat broth thickened with yam and tomato.
● Mashed fresh fish with vegetable stew.
● Finely minced liver with yam or rice.

Add to all these ¼ teaspoon of fat or edible oil.

And pineapple or orange juice, paw paw or mashed banana.

Evening
Cereal with milk or half boiled egg (if baby has not had it in the morning), or mashed banana and milk.

So, at 6–9 months the baby should be eating daily

Body building foods
● Groundnuts.
● Beans.
● Fish.
● Meat.
● Eggs.

Energy giving foods
● Milk.
● Fat or edible oil.
● Cereal or yam or sweet potato.

Protective foods
● Green and yellow vegetables.
● Fruit juices or mashed fruit.

The baby at 9–12 months
The baby still needs food *specially prepared* even though the actual items of food are the same as the grown ups are eating.

But remember – no spicy or hot foods.

Breakfast
Choose one of the following
● Cereal with milk.
● Cereal with a local bean preparation for children.
● Egg added to the gruel.
● Banana mashed in milk.

Lunch
Any of the following
● Mashed yam, green vegetable with minced meat. Add a little fat or oil.
● Rice, green vegetable with minced meat.
● Yam, tomato, palm oil and finely chopped liver.
● *Or* Same as above with fish instead of meat.
● Beans and rice stew with added oil.
● Bean stew.
● Mashed beans.

244

- Groundnut soup, boiled rice.
- Groundnut stew.
- Plantain porridge with groundnuts, meat or fish in the sauce.

Afternoon
Fruit

Evening
Give something which the baby hasn't already had, such as one of the following
- Cereal with pounded crayfish or groundnuts.
- Beans and rice.
- Lightly boiled egg and bread.
- Plantain porridge.
  With milk to drink – or fruit.

Diet for a baby 1–2 years old

Breakfast
Gruel and milk with special bean preparation. *Or* Bread, butter, milk and half boiled egg.

Lunch
Groundnut stew or bone and marrow soup with one of the following
- Yam pottage, with meat and/or fish.
- Beans and rice stew or beans and yam stew.
- Vegetable stew with fish or chopped meat.
- Rice and beans with meat stew.
- Bean and plantain stew.
- Plantain pottage or porridge with any vegetable and meat or fish.
- Thick porridge made from maize or cassava flour with soup made from oil, fish, okro and green leaf.

Afternoon
Fruit in season such as orange, banana, pineapple, paw paw.

Supper

Banana.

Or Pap with banana.

Or Mashed yam with beans or egg.

Or Bread and milk with half boiled egg.

Or Plantain or softly boiled rice with vegetable stew — with fish or chopped meat when possible.

Diet for a 2–5 year old

Breakfast

Pap with fried yam.

Or Cereal and a bean preparation.

Or Bread and butter and egg.

Lunch

Best if it has three items **Triple Mix**

1   **Staple**: yam — rice — or cassava, maize or plantain.
2   **Vegetable**: stew from green leaf, okro, tomato, onion, egusi with palm oil or groundnut oil.
3   **Protein**: meat, liver or fish, beans or groundnuts made into stew with stock from marrow and bones.

Afternoon

Fruits in season such as banana, oranges, mangoes, guava, paw paw and pineapple.

Supper

Again, if possible, Triple Mix.

A **staple** like rice, 'garri', cassava, yam, corn, millet, plantain, with a **body building food** like egg, fish, groundnuts or beans — and **vegetables** in season.

Also fruits in season.

Note $\frac{1}{2}$–1 egg daily. Meat 2–3 times a week and on other days fish. This of course depends on whether the family live near a river or if fish is obtainable.

246

3 Advising on diets for specific deficiencies

Table 19.2 *Nutrient content of common tropical foods*

Nutrient	Daily Requirement M. (20–29 yrs.)	F. (20–29 yrs.)	Child (1–3 yrs.)	FOOD SOURCE and approximate nutritive value (in units given below each nutrient in col. 1) per 100 g (3½ oz) of edible portion			
Protein (g)	70	65	40	Whole milk	18	Fish, fresh	3
				Dried milk	60	Fish, dry	30
				Offal	20	Pulses (peas, beans, etc.)	18
				Egg	35	Soya beans	13
				Meat	27	Groundnuts	18
				Cheese	8	Cereals	20
Calories	2850	2150	1300	Oils	900	Pulses	340
				Butter, lard	750	Cereals	350
				Oil seeds, groundnuts	580	Starchy roots and fruits	110
Calcium (mg)	500	400	400	Whole milk	100	Beans and peas	120
				Evaporated milk	1500	Sesame seeds	300
				Dried milk	250	Dark green leaves (e.g. spinach)	1000
				Cheese (hard)	3000	Dried fish (in which bones are eaten)	800
				Soya beans	200		
				Whole finger millet	350		

Table 19.2 (contd.)

Nutrient	M. (20–29 yrs.)	Daily Requirement F. (20–29 yrs.)	Child (1–3 yrs.)	FOOD SOURCE and approximate nutritive value (in units given below each nutrient in col. 1) per 100 g (3½ oz) of edible portion			
Iron (mg)	13	15	9	Liver	10	Dark green leaves	3
				Kidney	10	Mid-green leaves (e.g. cassava, pumpkin)	3
				Heart	4	Millet	3
				Meat	3	Sorghum	4
				Fish, dry	8	Maize flour	2
				Eggs	3	Oil seeds	5–10
				Yeast	20	Cashew, pumpkin, sesame seeds	10
				Lake fly	66	Beans, peas	5–9
Vitamin A (i.u.)	4800	4400	2000	Liver	20,000	Dark green leaves	3000
				Kidney	1,000	Mid-green leaves	1000
				Egg	1,000	Carrots	3000
				Butter	3,000	Pumpkins	350
				Animal ghee	2,000	Mangoes	600
				Cheese	1,400	Paw paws	1000
				Fortified margarine oil and ghee	3,000	Cooking bananas	100
				Whole dried milk	1,200	Sweet potatoes	100
				Fish liver oil	100,000	Jak fruit	150
				Red palm oil	20,000	Yellow maize	150

248

Nutrient	Daily Requirement M. F. (20–29 yrs.)	Child (1–3 yrs.)	FOOD SOURCE and approximate nutritive value (in units given below each nutrient in col. 1) per 100 g (3½oz) of edible portion			
Thiamin (mg)	1	0.6	Maize, whole	0.4	Lake fly	1.2
			Low extract millet whole	0.3	Beans, peas	5–9
			Millet flour	0.2	Soya beans	1.1
			Sorghum whole	0.5	Oil seeds, e.g.	0.9
			Sorghum flour	0.4	groundnuts, cashew	0.6
			Rice unpolished	0.3	sesame, sunflower	1.0
			Yeast, brewers	9.5	Liver, heart, kidney	0.4
			Sorghum beer	0.2	Milk powder	0.4
Riboflavin (mg)	1.5 1.3	0.9	Whole milk	0.2	Pulses	0.2
			Dried milk	1.3	Soya beans	0.3
			Cheese	0.4	Oil seeds	0.2
			Liver	2.5	Dark green leaves	0.3
			Kidney	2.0	Mid green leaves	0.2
			Meat	0.2	Mushrooms	0.5
			Maize whole	0.1		
			Millet whole	0.1		
			Sorghum whole	0.1		

Table 19.2 (contd.)

Nutrient	Daily Requirement			FOOD SOURCE and approximate nutritive value (in units given below each nutrient in col. 1) per 100 g (3½oz) of edible portion	
	M.	F.	Child		
	(20–29 yrs.)		(1–3 yrs.)		
Niacin (mg)	14	12	6	Liver	13.0
				Kidney, heart	7.0
				Meat	5.0
				Chicken	9.0
				Maize	1.0
				Millet	1.0
				Rice	1.0
				Sorghum	3.5
				Fish, fresh	2.0
				Fish, dry	6.0
				Beans and peas	2.0
				Groundnuts	17.0
				Sesame and sunflower seeds	5.0
				Mushrooms	6.0
				Yeast	30.0
Vitamin C (g)	25	25	20	Dark green leaves	100
				Other green leaves	45
				Citrus fruit	40
				Oranges, tangerines	
				Paw paws	50
				Guavas	200
				Baobab pulp	370
				Mangoes, pineapples	30
				Liver	30
				Fresh cassava	30
				Bananas	20
				Sweet potatoes	30

CHAPTER 20

Fluids Used in Nasogastric Tube Feeding

Used

● **As total intake** in some instances.
- Tetanus when child unable to swallow at all.
- Unconsciousness, e.g. after head injury.
● **To supplement oral feeding** when child not taking *enough*.
- Patients with poor appetite e.g. typhoid.
- Malnutrition.
- Convalescent tetanus.

Requirements

● Consistency − should be able to run through tube easily.
● Ideal concentration 1 kcal/ml.
● Simple formula so it can be made up in ward.
● Make 24 hours requirement and keep in fridge until used.
● Fat should not be more than 35% kcal.

Give

● 3 hourly or 4 hourly. Rest at night, e.g. If 4 hourly give at 6 a.m. − 10 a.m. − 2 p.m. − 6 p.m. − 10 p.m.
● Run in by gravity.
● Typical feeding schedule starting with dilute feeds is shown in Table 20.1.

Table 20.1

Day	Type of feed	Daily amount	Divided into
1	$\frac{1}{2}$ strength milk feeds	150 ml/kg body weight	12 feeds/day
2	$\frac{1}{2}$ strength milk feeds	150 ml/kg body weight	8 feeds/day
3 and 4	$\frac{2}{3}$ strength milk feeds	150 ml/kg body weight	8 feeds/day
5 onwards	Full strength milk feeds	150 ml/kg body weight	6 feeds/day

● Vitamin supplement necessary daily.

Principles

Kilocalorie requirement
1000 at 1 year, and 100 for each extra year up to 12, e.g. 7 year old needs 1700 kcal.

Protein and fluid requirements
See in Table 20.2.

Table 20.2

Age in years	Protein g/kg/day	If weight unknown protein in g	Fluid req. ml/kg
0–1	2	20	150
1–3	1.5	25	100
3–6	1.25	30	90
7–12	1.0	40	70
18	0.5–1.0	45	50

Total number of grams of protein required multiplied by 4 = number of calories obtained from protein.

Fat
Not more than 35% of total calorie requirement.
Number of calories as fat divided by 9 = grams of fat.

Carbohydrate
Give remaining calories as carbohydrate.
Number of remaining calories divided by 4 = grams of carbohydrate (CHO).

Alternative mixtures
Using either of 2 mixtures shown in Table 20.3 and 20.4, calculating by calorie requirement only, the protein, fat and carbohydrate concentration will be satisfactory.

252

Table 20.3   1000 ml 1000 calories

	Amount g oz	Protein g	Fat g	CHO g
Complan	90 3	28	14	40
Evaporated milk	120 4	9	10	15
Oil	15 ½	–	15	–
Glucose	75 2½	–	–	68
Water to	1000	37	39	123

Table 20.4   1000 ml 1000 calories

	Amount g	Protein g	Fat g	CHO g
Complan	100	31	16	44
Evaporated milk	80	6	7	10
Oil	15	–	15	–
Glucose	80	–	–	72
Water to	1000	37	38	126

● But if Complan and evaporated milk not available use the mixture shown in Table 20.5.

Table 20.5   1000 ml 800 calories

	Amount g	Protein g	Fat g	CHO g
Casilan	30	27	0.6	–
Dried skimmed milk	33	10.6	5.3	13
Glucose	75	–	–	68
Oil	45	–	30	–
Water to	1000	37.6	35.9	81

(This has 40% of calories as fat and should only be used for a few days.)
● If evaporated milk is available use the mixture shown in Table 20.6.

Table 20.6   1000 ml 840 calories (also higher fat content)

	Amount g	Protein g	Fat g	CHO g
Casilan	30	27	0.6	–
Evaporated milk	120	9.4	10.1	14.8
Oil	30	–	30	–
Glucose	75	–	–	68.3
Water to	1000	38.4	40.7	83.1

● *High energy feed*

Table   20.7

	Milk ml g	Oil ml	Sugar ml
Cow's/goat's milk	900	60	80
*Skimmed milk powder	90	95	75
*Full cream milk powder	120	60	75
*Evaporated milk	430	55	80
K-MIX 2 reconstituted	130 120	95	40

*After mixing with oil and sugar, make up to 1000 ml with water.

Energy value 1350–1360 kcal per 1000 ml fluid.
+K-MIX 2 – see below.
● *Alternatively* tablespoons and cups (250 ml) may be used.

Table 20.8

	Milk	Oil (tbsp)	Sugar (tbsp)
Cow's/goat's milk	3¾ cups	5	7
Skimmed milk powder	13 tbsp	8	7
Full cream milk powder	15 tbsp	5	7
Evaporated milk	1¾ cups	5	6
K-MIX 2 unreconstituted	10 tbsp	8	4

1 tbsp = 15 ml or 12.5 g sugar
1 cup = 250 ml or 208 g sugar
Energy value 1350–1360 kcal per 1000 ml
          or 135–136 kcal per 100 ml.

- *To prepare* If using milk powder — mix with sugar and oil to a smooth paste. Then add to it small quantities of warm — not hot — water that has been boiled and cooled. Mix with an egg beater. If using an electric blender all the ingredients can be blended together. If using fluid milk an electric blender or rotary egg beater may be used. Clean very well after each use.
- $^+$K-MIX 2 — a food mixture distributed by UNICEF.
Mix 100 g of K-MIX 2 with 50 g (58 ml) of vegetable oil to a smooth paste. Gradually add 1 litre of water stirring well. If the vegetable oil separates on standing, stir briskly before feeding. The composition of K-MIX 2 is shown in Table 20.9.

Table 20.9

Calcium caseinate	3 parts by weight
Skimmed milk powder	5 parts by weight
Sucrose	10 parts by weight
Retinol palmitate	5,000 i.u. Vitamin A per 100 g dry mixture

Vitamins
Vitamins are advisable when a child is fed by nasogastric tube and not taking ordinary diet. Give a multi-vitamin preparation daily through the N.G. tube.

K-MIX 2 is of value as it contains Vitamin A. In those areas where palm oil is available — and also if the child can tolerate it — use as an excellent source of Vitamin A.

Useful Figures Constituents in g/100 g

Table 20.10

/100 g	Protein	Fat	Carbohydrate	Calories
Casilan	90	1.8	—	450
Complan	31	16	44 (includes lactose)	450
Evaporated milk	7.8	8.4	12.3	120
Dried skimmed milk	31.2	16	40	428
Glucose	—	—	91	364
Edible oil	—	100	—	900

● CHAPTER 21

Health Education

● Health education is as important as medical and nursing care. In the daily ward schedule time should be set aside for health education. A senior and experienced person amongst the ward team is the ideal person to organise the sessions. The more junior staff should be encouraged to assist so that they can learn the necessary techniques.

A useful principle to bear in mind is:

> 'What we hear we forget.
> What we see we remember.
> But what we do we know.'

● Hence, make the sessions as practical as possible. To make the sessions relevant always start with one of the participants asking a question or giving a small talk.
● When children are discharged from the hospital, encourage the parents to come back. A parents' club may be started in this way. Some of the more active parents who have seen their children recover may become regular speakers and relate their experiences.
● Avoid the temptation to use sophisticated audio-visual aids like slides, films, tape recorders or video cassettes. More can be understood by the teacher and the learner through a short one-to-one exchange, or through group discussions than by such impersonal aids. The best audio-visual aid is involvement in activity.
● Avoid introducing too many complex ideas in one session. Build each session round one main theme or objective. Look for imaginative ways of introducing the theme involving the participants as much as possible and always include an activity instead of having the participants listening passively.

Some practical suggestions

● Have a list of subjects and keep a record of:
– the date;
– group spoken to;
– title of talk.
  Otherwise you give the same 2–3 talks all the time and people 'turn you off' like the radio.
● Use the local language where possible and especially local names for diseases.
● Invite mothers to ask questions – and never laugh at questions or regard them as foolish.
● Before starting a talk, ask who was there at the last one. Ask them questions about it.
● In cooking demonstrations use local cooking utensils and local means of cooking, e.g. do not use electric cookers. If cooking is on open fires at home, then aim to demonstrate using an open fire, or a charcoal burner. Use as few utensils as possible since most homes make do with a few pots and stirring spoons.

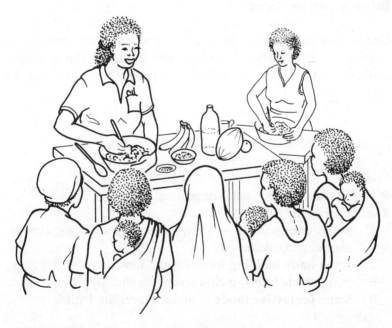

Cooking demonstration

Talk 1 How to keep well during pregnancy and have a healthy baby

The concept

The care of the child begins at conception. Because for the first 9 months of its life the baby is not accessible, the care is to be provided through the care of the mother.

Special clinics for checking the health of the pregnant woman have been set up. Here the health workers make sure that there are no illnesses in the mother, the baby is growing well, and medicines for the protection of the mother and the baby are given.

The mothers themselves can do a great deal to ensure the health of the baby by eating well, not over-exerting, especially in the later stages of pregnancy, and, in general, by following the advice given at the clinic.

Introducing the concept

One or two mothers may be asked to relate their experiences in pregnancy. If possible a mother who attended the antenatal clinic should be asked to relate her experience of attending the clinic.

Points to stress

Food

● Eat 3 meals a day – not 2 huge ones.
● Remember the rule of 3.
  1 Some **energy** food – yam, garri, rice or other cereals, plantain, cocoyam, oil.
  2 Some **body building** food (for the new baby) – fish, egg, milk, meat, beans, melon seeds, crayfish or groundnuts.
  3 Some **protective foods** – green vegetable, fruits.

Serve a little extra on your plate **for the baby**.

Exercise
- Don't sit all day — and don't *stand* all day.
- Carry on with your usual routine.

Rest
- Lie down and rest 8 hours at night. It is also good to lie down for 1–2 hours in the middle of the day.

Antenatal clinic
- Always attend an antenatal clinic at a maternity clinic or hospital and you will get advice and help there. Begin as soon as you know that you are pregnant.
- Take the Sunday Sunday medicine (antimalarial) to prevent malaria. Malaria stops the baby from growing, or even makes him come too soon before he is strong.
- Take any other treatment they give you e.g. the tablets to build up your blood.
- Do not take any tablets bought from the market or anywhere else — they may do the baby harm. Only the necessary tablets are given from the clinic and these will not harm but help the growing baby.
- Do not take injections from other people either at home, in the market or anywhere else. At the clinic ask for the injection to protect your baby from tetanus — a condition which causes spasms and always kills.
- If you are continually sick, or having headaches, or having swelling of ankles or anywhere else, or bleeding, or leaking, or if you discover that the baby is not moving inside you, report to the nurse, clinic or hospital. These are danger signals.

Delivery
- Deliver in a place where a properly trained person can help you — that means a trained nurse or midwife or a birth attendant — in a clinic or hospital. Make sure that skilled help is available at all times if needed.
- If you deliver at home there is more chance of:
- difficulties in labour;
- infection for yourself and the baby;
- the baby not being strong and robust when it is born;
- the baby getting tetanus.

Talk 2   Care of the newborn baby

The concept

The main needs of the newborn are: warmth, food, love and protection from infection. If the baby is breast fed and nursed in the same bed as the mother he is getting all the first 3 and to a large extent protection from infection as well.

A great deal of harm can be caused by certain practices like applying various preparations to the cord stump, giving enemas and purges, and circumcision by untrained persons.

Introducing the talk

A trained village midwife may be able to recount what she normally advises. Alternatively, the participants may start with a discussion on what practices are generally followed in the community.

Points to stress

Feeding
- It is good to feed the baby quite soon after delivery if the baby is crying or wants to suck.
- From then on most mothers know 'by nature' when to feed their babies. Therefore it is good to have the baby in a cot near you so you can pick her up when you want to.
- The breast milk is watery for the first 2−3 days but this is natural, and is special for babies at this age. Do not worry if it looks yellow. That is how it is meant to be.
- Do not give tinned milk at this time.
- Do not use a feeding bottle **ever**.
- Breast milk is best.
- If a mother is really sick the nurses should feed the baby with a **cup and spoon**.

Be prepared
- Have a few dresses, nappies, towels and face cloth for the new baby.

● Have a *place* for the baby to sleep in. Some can afford a cot, others a box lined with clean cloths.

Washing
● Start with the face and hands and work down to the legs.

Eyes
● Do not put anything into the eyes.
● Eyelids can be wiped with the baby's damp face cloth.

Cord
● In some hospitals dressings are applied to the end of the cord. This is to stop people from putting milk, oil, spiders web, clay or home remedies on it. But it is better if **no covering** is on the cord. It will dry up and fall off on its own.

Circumcision
Hundreds of babies die each year following tetanus from native circumcision. Get your baby circumcised in hospital or clinic.

Purges and enemas
These are often given as home remedies — and they can **kill babies**. If the baby is sick, bring him to a nurse in the clinic.

Talk 3   Young babies crying too much

The concept

Responding to the needs of the baby is an important part of parenthood. Babies express needs, discomfort or pain through crying. By anticipating needs and by avoiding discomfort a mother can help a baby grow with a happy disposition. Sometimes, however, excessive or incessant crying may indicate an illness.

Introducing the concept

Get the mothers to talk about what they do to comfort their babies when they cry. There may be a number of beliefs related to crying in the newborn period. Get the mothers to talk about them if you can.

Points to stress

Cause may be simple.
- Too hot – too many clothes on, e.g. a bonnet in the hot season.
- Or cold – in the rainy season at night.
- Or wet – needs clothes changing.
- Or hungry – especially babies who are *not* breast fed.
- Or wanting love – mother is out working, and person looking after the child doesn't pick her up. Or perhaps even mother doesn't hold the baby enough.
- Or a habit – of breast feeding on and off all night. When mother decides to stop – baby cannot sleep.
- Or when weaning – from the breast – too suddenly.

But if there is no obvious reason **and crying continues** remember it may be
- Earache – due to inflammation of the ear.
- Bellyache
- because someone gave purge or enema;
- or because mother didn't get the wind up after feed.
- Or, in newborns – it may be an early sign of **tetanus** and other troubles.

So *if it continues* get an expert to see – take child to the children's clinic.

Prevent the crying by
- Getting the wind up after a feed. That is holding the baby upright and patting the back.
- When the baby is older and you are changing from breast feeding to cup feeding, do it very gradually over 4 weeks, not *suddenly*.

Talk 4   Injections and medicine to prevent children getting diseases

The concept

A number of childhood illnesses are preventable by immunisations. Developing measles or whooping cough is not part of the growing up process as believed by some. Nor does it toughen the child. On the contrary these are dangerous illnesses. Even if the child were to recover, there are risks of complications or various disabilities, as in the case of poliomyelitis.

Introducing the concept

Ask the parents to recall their own experiences as children when they had measles. Do they know of any deaths following measles? Do they know of any child in the neighbourhood or community who is lame? How did it happen?

Points to stress

● So many babies' and children's illnesses can be prevented.
● Which ones?
  – TB
  – Diphtheria
  – Tetanus
  – Whooping cough
  – Measles
  – Poliomyelitis (use local names)
● The baby will be so much stronger if she grows up *without* these sicknesses.
● *When* should a baby be *immunised*? Some are given at birth and some others at various ages between birth and 9 months.
● Parents cannot remember all these things so it will be written on the child's *weight card*.
● Do they last for life? No – you need repeat doses for some of them at 18 months and 5 years. For this, further appointments will be made at the clinic.

- If a child didn't get them at the right time, is it too late? No, it is never too late to start.
- Can a child get measles or whooping cough after vaccination? Yes, sometimes that can happen. But mostly the infants are protected by vaccination.
- *When* can a parent get these services? Ask at the local clinic. Or give out the details.

    At *this* clinic we give (... ... ...)

Talk 5   Giving a drink of water

The concept

Small infants do not need additional water, even in very hot weather. Breast milk is enough. So there is no need to give a glucose or sugar drink to the baby. The older children need a drink of water now and again. But never use feeding bottles, nor force-feed by hand.

Introducing the concept

Get the mothers to talk about what they normally do. What is the source of their water supply? If not piped water, do they boil it? How is the water stored in the home? How does the baby drink: from a feeding bottle? a cup? force-feeding by hand?

Points to stress

- Small babies up to 3−4 months do not need additional water to drink if you have plenty of breast milk.
- After that, especially in the hot season, they do need it − but it has to be **clean** and given in the right way.
- For the water to be safe to drink, boil it and allow it to cool, and store in a clean white bottle (not a brown one that you cannot see into). Cork it well. Boiling kills the germs of diarrhoea.
- Give it with cup and spoon − at first. Later by cup. Keep a special cup and spoon for the baby which are 'scalded' with boiling water before use each time in order to kill any germs.

- **Do not use feeding bottles** – germs live inside them and cause diarrhoea and vomiting.
- **Do not use force-feeding by hand.** First, because there may be germs on the hand (and you cannot boil your hand like you can a cup). Secondly, because the water rushes in the mouth and may go down the wrong way and choke the baby. A baby can die because of this.

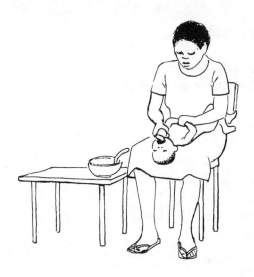

Do not force feed

- **Do not hold the baby upside down to feed** as they do in some areas. Why – because every week some babies **drown** when the water goes the wrong way and they cannot get air.
- If a baby is ill and does not want to drink – or refuses – do not force him – you may choke him. Bring him to see a doctor, a nurse or a midwife who will examine the baby and advise you.
- When children have fever or are sick they usually need *more* water – so remember to give them drinks more often.

Most important **Never use feeding bottles or hands to feed.** So many babies have died from these and the mothers haven't known why.

Talk 6 Cleanliness

The concept

Cleanliness in the home and personal hygiene provide a healthy environment for the babies to grow in. Clean food and water help to avoid diarrhoea. If the surroundings of the house are kept clean there will be fewer flies and mosquitoes.

Introducing the subject

Practical demonstrations with participation by the mothers and using pictures if available are most effective.

Points to stress

Cleanliness of
1 The baby or child.
2 The clothes.
3 Drinking water − milk − food.
4 The surroundings.

The baby or child
● Newborns need not be bathed. Infants and older children need a daily bath. Clean the face, armpits and genitalia gently with soap and water. Rinse with water.
● Start at the head and work down.
● In the wet season wash and dry quickly. Do not allow to get cold.
● Do not let soapy water get into the eyes or mouth.
● Keep nails short, not long and dirty.
● Wash your hands after going to the latrine or after cleaning up the baby's stool.

Clothes
● Wash and dry on a line. Don't leave on the ground for the tumbo fly to lay eggs in them and cause abcesses in the baby.

Drinking water – milk – food

● Don't give water or any food item by hand. The hand may not be free of germs.
● Don't give baby water straight from a stream.
● Boil the baby's water. Cool and store in a clean bottle with cork.
● *Never* use a feeding bottle. Diarrhoea germs hide inside the teats.
● Cover all food – wash all fruit.
● Wash hands before eating.

Surroundings

● Keep the house and compound clean, and teach the children to do this too.
● Bury or burn refuse.
● If you have a bin, use a tight-fitting lid.
● Ask your local government to get pipe-borne water if you haven't got it yet.
● If you use a well – keep it covered.

Talk 7   Under-five weight charts

The concept

A good sign of health is that the baby is growing well. We measure growth by weighing the child, by measuring the increase in length or height and by measuring the thickness or fatness (circumference) of the limbs. In order to make sure that the baby is growing from month to month or from year to year we need to maintain a record. This is known as the Road to Health Chart. We also enter records of illnesses, immunisations and other details on this card. Thus, it is a very important piece of paper. Every time the child is taken to the clinic the card should be brought along to update the health information on it.

Introducing the concept

Practical demonstrations of weighing, and recording on a weight chart are essential. Flannelgraphs are ideal for teaching. Mothers should understand the significance of 'Road to Health' and should be taught the interpretation of the weight curve.

Points to stress

- Passport to health.
- Death and illness are preventable.
- Show the path to good health.
- If child is *off* the path there is likely to be danger to his health.
- Regular weighing is essential to judge how the baby is growing.
- If *on* the path – we must strive to keep the baby there.
- If *off* the path – we must help the baby to get on again.
- Attend monthly for regular checking of weight.
- Immunisations are also recorded on the weight chart.
- *Keep* the card safe and *bring* it every time you attend the clinic with the child.

Discuss the following

- Like passports – if you carry one of these cards for your child he can be helped to grow on the road to health.
- Babies and children *don't* have to die and get so many illnesses.
- On this card is the path to health (show with finger). This path shows the weight, and we mark the weight every month from birth to 5 years.
- When the weight is off the path to health, the baby is sick, or is going to be sick. Once we know this we can *do* something or *prevent* a risk to the baby's life.
- We can only do this if the baby is brought to the Under 5's Clinic regularly and weighed.
- If the baby is on the path to health, the health workers will help you to keep him there; that is by preventing malaria measles, diarrhoea and other disease, and by proper diet.
- If the baby is off the path, the health workers will also tell you how to get him onto it again.
- So come *at least* monthly until the baby is 2 years old and 2 monthly afterwards and any time that the baby is not well.
- The health workers will also record immunisations on this card – so wherever you go there will be a record.
- **Keep this card safe – and bring it every time you come to the clinic. All the family details entered on the card are safe with you because you keep the card. Do not lose it.**

Talk 8   Feeding

The concept

Babies and young children can be fed adequately from locally available foods. Many of them can be easily grown in the back garden. The child's stomach is small, and the requirements to satisfy growth are high. So children need to be fed more often than adults. Secondly, the small quantities a child eats at each mealtime should give him plenty of energy. Hence, add a small amount of oil or fat to each meal. This is particularly so during illness and convalescence.

Introducing the concept

Start a discussion going by asking what makes babies grow. Why are they weak after an illness? What foods are best for babies? Demonstrate the local foods. Ask for the prices. Ask which foods can be grown in the back garden. Which foods the mothers can afford to buy.

Points to stress

The 3 kinds of food
1   Those that **give energy**.
   – Yam, rice, 'garri', plantain, banana, palm oil, groundnut oil and sugar.

2   Those that **build the body and keep it strong**.
   – Mother's milk, other milks, fish, meat, eggs, beans, groundnuts, melon seeds, crayfish.

3   Those that **protect the body** from sickness.
   – Fruits and vegetables, especially green vegetables, and yellow fruits like paw paw and oranges.

To stay well and to grow well, we need the rule of 3.
Give your children and yourself 3 meals a day.
Each meal should have something from all the 3 groups.

Talk 9 Breast feeding

The concept

Breast feeding is best for the baby
- because it is the milk *especially made* for babies (milk in tins is prepared from cow's milk which is meant for calves).
- because breast fed babies *don't get so many illnesses* as those who are not breast fed. Breast milk contains protective substances to *protect* the baby.
- because breast feeding helps the growth of the *whole* baby, the body as well as the mind and feelings. Babies who are breast fed experience their mothers' love to the full, in the close contact during suckling.

Introducing the concept

Get a discussion going with the statement *'Some mothers bottle feed their babies. Why?'*

Usual answers given are
- I see everyone doing it now.
- You can get bottles in the market.
- I go out to work.
- It's better for the baby, isn't it?

Emphasise that
- 'Everyone' doesn't necessarily do the best thing. Very often one's own culture and traditions are best. In this case it is very true. Even countries who export feeding bottles and dried milk have realised their mistake and are going back to breast feeding themselves now.
- Many of you used to go to work when you had babies before and *also* breast fed. If you have to miss a feed while you are working — you can still breast feed the rest of the time. Arrange for the baby to have dried milk and water mixture by **cup** or **cup and spoon** when you are away.
- Dried milk is *not* better for babies than breast milk. Human mother's milk is best for the human baby. Why? See if you remember what has just been said.

270

Common results of bottle feeding

- Many mothers may know how to sterilise a feeding bottle, but when they go out and leave the baby in the care of someone else — any of the following may happen.
- The feed is not finished and the bottle is left standing — flies settle on the teat. Diarrhoea germs carried on the legs of the flies infect the teat — soon the baby has loose stools.
- As the baby gets older, insufficient milk powder is put in the water — baby soon loses weight and gets thin.
- Other mothers live far from the stream — water is in short supply — they don't know how to sterilise the bottle and teat. Take the teat off and look on the inside. Old milk and dirt are ideal for germs to multiply.
- Baby has diarrhoea over and over again.
- Thousands **die each year**.
- Powdered milk is expensive and it is tempting to economise by using less of the powder. This means that the baby is getting watery milk and babies cannot grow on water. So they become thin and wasted.

Do you agree? Who is going to throw away the bottle or give it to me now? **Then you can feed baby on the breast** or with a **cup** and have a healthier, happier baby.

Talk 10 Purges and enemas

The concept

Giving frequent purges and enemas to babies and young children is a harmful practice.

Introducing the concept

Start a discussion with the statement 'It has been our tradition to give purges and enemas, but now we know they can do much harm'. Continue by introducing the following topics into the discussion.

What harm?
- They can cause distended abdomen.

- Perforation of intestine and death.
- Some substances used as purges or enemas can poison the baby.
- Some substances are good for one use, e.g. cleaning toilets — but not meant for the inside of a baby e.g. Izal, Dettol.
- Some substances do not harm adults but can kill babies, e.g. castor oil. There is violent diarrhoea causing loss of water from the body.
- Prolapse of anus, because the nozzle of the enema tube is too big for the baby.

How many times a day should a baby pass a stool?
We are all different. Some go 2–3 times a day. Some go once a day — that is good. Sometimes it is once in 2 days — that is also good.

What can keep the stool from being too hard?
Young infants can take mashed fruits and older ones green leaf and vegetables. Then everything is all right. That is what nature planned for us to keep us well.

If a baby cries — doesn't it mean he needs to pass a stool and cannot?
No — it can mean many things.
- Wind.
- Hunger — or even the opposite — overfeeding.
- Wet napkin.
- Wanting love.
- Insect bite.
- Tired of lying in one position.
- Thirsty.

So when baby cries
- Check if he is dry or wet and give a drink or food if necessary. With small babies, help them to bring the wind up after each feed so it won't stay there and cause pain.

To prevent crying
- Breast feed (not bottle).
- Give enough *rest* — don't hold him all day and all evening — allow him to lie down at times.

272

- See if he is dry and needs a drink.
- Get the wind up after each feed.
- Give him love and talk or sing to him.
- Attend the child welfare clinic and get weight checked monthly.

- If you do all this, and the baby is crying, he may be sick or he may have an earache, so take the baby to clinic or hospital for the nurse to see.
- There is far more diarrhoea and vomiting here than in other countries. Why? Partly because of feeding bottles and partly because of purges and enemas.
- Instead of weekly purge give weekly **Sunday Sunday Medicine** and stop malaria fever − then your child will be strong.
- Instead of monthly enema **go to clinic** and get immunisation against measles, whooping cough and other sickness.

Talk 11   Fever

The concept

Fever is one of the commonest signs of illness in a child. In malarial areas malaria is the commonest cause. Respiratory infections and diarrhoea may also cause fever. Measles and other similar illnesses also begin with fever.

Dangers
- The fever may be a sign of an illness starting, e.g. measles or severe cough, although the commonest is **malaria**.
- Some children tend to get **convulsions** when they get fever from any cause.

Introducing the concept

Ask what can be done to prevent fever. End up by stressing prevention.

Prevention
Prevent fever by having a healthy child, and you do this by attending Under-5 Clinic or Children's Clinic regularly.

Have you got
- antimalaria tablets to prevent malaria?
- immunisations and vaccination to prevent measles and other conditions causing fever?

Go on to discuss the following points.

When your child develops fever
● The most likely cause is **malaria** so we will talk a lot about this now.
● If the fever continues after treatment for malaria is given, there must be another cause, e.g. measles, pneumonia. See a nurse or bring the child to the clinic.

Malaria

Harmful effects
● Causes fever, anaemia, poor appetite, loss of weight, enlarged spleen, possibly convulsions, and kills thousands of children each year.
● Makes pregnant women start labour and have their babies before time − so they are small or weak.

Cause
The **mosquito** which carries the malaria from one person to another.

Prevention
● Stop mosquitoes multiplying by:
- keeping the compound clean and flat, so there are no pools of water;
- burying unwanted tins and containers;
- covering water pots and any other place where there is water.
● Give children antimalarials (Sunday Sunday medicine) regularly until 5 years old.
● Attend Under-5 clinic or Children's Clinic where you may obtain the antimalarials.

If fever starts
● Treatment for malaria is **chloroquine**. Find out the dose for *your* child in the clinic and keep some tablets at home.

● Start treatment and bring the child to the clinic if not improving in a few hours. Never give more than the dose recommended.

Talk 12   Diarrhoea and vomiting

The concept

Diarrhoea is one of the major killer diseases of children in the developing world. It is preventable. When it does occur, quick intervention in the home with the sugar/salt solution will avoid severe complications.

Introducing the concept

Ask the mothers how many of their children have suffered from diarrhoea? Do they know of any deaths in the neighbourhood from diarrhoea? What do people normally do as treatment? What do they know about prevention?

Points to stress

Prevention at the community level
● Try and get pipe-borne water so you *can* keep child, self and house clean and get clean water to drink.

What mothers and families can do for their children
● Breast feed only from birth to 4 or 5 months. No tinned milk. No feeding bottle. No hand feeding − not even cereal.
● At 4−5 months *continue* breast feeding. This helps to fight diarrhoea. Also give other foods by cup and spoon.
● No feeding bottles ever. Germs which cause diarrhoea hide inside the teat. Use cup and spoon.
● Boil all water for the baby − cool and store in clear glass bottle with top.
● Clean linen. Keep surroundings and child clean. Wash child's hands before eating and after going to the latrine.
● Keep the food covered. Wash fruit before eating or peeling.
● Enemas and purges cause loose frequent stools − so *stop* them.

- Malaria causes diarrhoea. So give the Sunday Sunday medicine weekly until the child is 5 years old.
- Prevent babies passing stool on the floor. Use nappies when smaller. Have proper latrine.
- Burn or bury refuse. If you have a bin, use a tight fitting lid. Refuse attracts flies and flies carry diarrhoea germs on their legs.

If baby gets diarrhoea
If no fever and is not looking sick.
- Give the baby water with sugar and salt made up as follows:
- a teaspoon of sugar;
- a 3-finger pinch of salt;
  to a mug of water which has been boiled and cooled.
- Give as much as the child will take. Prepare another mug as soon as one is finished.

You will prevent serious trouble if you do this.
- Watch the baby and stools.
- If diarrhoea is less and the stools becoming formed, repeat sugar/salt/water.
- But if stools continue to remain watery and frequent, or if baby is feverish or vomiting, then take a clinic or hospital urgently.

If baby is very hot, or is vomiting or if the soft place on baby's head goes down.
- Take baby to clinic or to a nurse or to hospital.

Cholera
Harmful effects are well known. Sudden onset of frequent watery stools, collapse and death if no emergency treatment is given.

Note There is a milder form where there is no collapse. This person may infect other people and children so it is important to prevent.

Prevention
- Do not pass stool into the stream or in the bush but have a proper latrine.

- Wash hands after going to latrine and before eating food.
- If cholera is in your area, boil drinking water if obtained from the stream.
- Wash fruit and vegetables.
- Keep plates and spoons clean.
- Cover food and water and destroy flies.

If child starts having frequent, watery stools.
- Give frequent drinks
- 1 teaspoon of sugar;
- a 3-finger pinch of salt;
- 1 mug of boiled, cooled water.
- If not improving, take to clinic at once.

Talk 13   Neonatal tetanus

The concept

Neonatal tetanus kills. After low birth weight it is the second most important cause of neonatal mortality in developing countries. It is also highly preventable through immunisation of the pregnant woman with the tetanus toxoid, and through clean cord handling after the birth of the baby. A great deal of neonatal tetanus stems from the local practice of applying various indigenous preparations to the cord stump.

Introducing the concept

- Ask about fits in the newborn period. What causes them? How to people treat fits in the newborn? How many babies die of them?
- Continue by using the vernacular name for tetanus.
- You know this sickness which makes babies:
- unable to suck, and they cry a lot at first;
- stiffen up and then have spasms;
- die in some days in spite of medical treatment.
- **The cause** is a germ (as in the case of diarrhoea). We cannot see it with our eye but it usually lives in dirt, earth, clay, sand, goat dung, ashes, limestone and cobwebs. When any of

these are applied to a cut or wound, the germ gains entry into the body and puts out its poison. The fits are caused by this poison.

● The **tetanus germ enters the body** through open wounds.
− Cut end of the cord.
− Circumcision wounds.
− Native scratches.
− Punching holes in the ear.
− Cutting of the uvula.
− Any wound.

Why do mothers apply things to the cord?
● In some places they believe the cord stump will drop off quicker and so the after pains will stop. This is false. **Leave the cord to dry up and drop off by itself.**
● **The after pains** are normal and are a sign that the uterus is becoming smaller, which it does in 10−14 days. It is something natural.

Advice
● Get antenatal care at a hospital or clinic. Get your 2 doses of tetanus vaccine while still pregnant.
● **Deliver** in a **clinic** or **hospital** (not at home or at a clinic run by an untrained person) because they know how to prevent tetanus.
● **Wherever** you **deliver**, do not apply anything to the cord − unless a nurse or doctor gives something special.
● **Allow it to dry up and fall off by itself** in 5−7 days.
● **If you have a male child**, get him circumcised at a clinic or hospital.
● **Keep all the baby's clothes** very clean and do not allow them to touch the ground.
● To **stop after pains** take some exercise every day and aspirin if the pain is worrying you.

Talk 14   Whooping cough and measles

The concept

Whooping cough and measles are both serious illnesses of

children. Both have a high mortality rate, and amongst those who recover there is a high risk of complications.

Introducing the concept

Ask the mothers if they have seen a child suffering from either of the two diseases. How do they recognise the illnesses? Are there other childhood illnesses that resemble them? Demonstrate the typical paroxysm of whooping cough.

Whooping cough

- Do the mothers know that small infants get whooping cough and often *die* from it, without ever *whooping*?
- Small babies
- get choked up and have thick mucus;
- sometimes go blue;
- later may cough (but not whoop); and may die.

Prevention
- Start your 3 in 1 immunisation, i.e. triple (or D.P.T.) which prevents whooping cough, as early as the clinic gives it, usually at 1 month.
- Attend for the 3-monthly injections for full protection and a booster at 18 months.
- If any child in your compound is whooping, keep your very young baby away from this child.

- **If your baby** is sick and you think he might have whooping cough, tell the nurse if there is someone else in the compound whooping. It is important they know.

- Best of all **prevent**.

Measles

Harmful effects
- Thousands of children die each year from this.
- Thousands of others become malnourished and in chronic ill-health following it.

279

● Many others are blinded, have chest trouble and other effects.

Prevention
● Have the child *immunised* against measles at the age of 9 months. This immunisation will not stop measles if the child has already got it (even though the rash has not yet appeared). So do not take the injection if the child has a fever – but tell the nurse and get advice.
● If there is no one giving measles immunisation in your area, mothers should get together, tell the Health Council and the Chiefs, and ask for it.

Note Do *not* take the child for immunisation if he/she has already *had* measles. It will not happen twice.

Talk 15   Convulsions

The concept

Convulsions are a common occurrence in children, often accompanying fever. The dangers usually arise from their management or the lack of it. Traditional methods of treatment like branding or giving cow's urine concoctions are dangerous. Without proper management recurrences with or without fever are common.

Convulsions are dangerous in the newborn period and in the first 6 months of life. Even in older children convulsions may be a sign of underlying serious disease. Hence in every case the child should be seen at the clinic.

Introducing the concept

Ask about what people think convulsions are due to. What are the popular methods of treatment? Do they know how to care for the child who is having a seizure?

Points to stress

● Convulsions are bad because of the possibility of damage to the child's *brain*.

Newborn babies
- **A seizure always signifies serious illness.**
- Avoid tetanus by taking immunisation during pregnancy and delivering in a proper maternity clinic or hospital.
- Don't apply *anything* to the cord — no sand or earth, etc. (Only if the nurse gives you a medicine for the purpose.)
- Get male babies circumcised in the clinic if you can.

Older babies and children
- Convulsions in a child less than 6 months old may be the first sign of a serious illness like meningitis. Rush him to the clinic or hospital.
- Malaria fever is the commonest cause. Prevent by giving Sunday Sunday medicine every week until the child is 5 years old.
- Any sickness with high fever can also cause convulsions. Attend the Under-5 Clinic to keep the child well.

What to do if the child (6 mths. – 5 yrs. old) has a convulsion with fever
- Keep calm — there is a lot you can do.
- Take off child's clothes and sponge all over with *cool* water.
- When convulsion stops, bring the child to the nearest clinic.
- If clinic is far away, give aspirin ($\frac{1}{4}-\frac{1}{2}$ tablet) with water when convulsion has stopped and when the child is *able to swallow without being forced*.
- **Don't** put the child in hot water or apply clay.
- **Don't** put pepper in the eyes or burn the legs.
- **Don't** *force* mouth open with a spoon, you can easily break the teeth.
- **Don't** give cow's urine medicine (which is done in some places) — it can cause brain damage.

Children who get convulsions every time they have a fever
- *Always* give antimalarial weekly.
- Ask in the clinic if you can have 5–10 tablets of aspirin, chloroquine and sedative tablets, so you can give some of each if the child develops convulsions in the night. You would give them *after* the convulsion. Find out the dose for *your* child. Be sure that you know it and will not make a mistake.

Children who have repeated convulsions and no fever
See a doctor — there is a special medicine that will stop these, but it must be taken *always* for 2 years.

Remember Convulsions cause brain damage. Convulsions can be prevented.

Talk 16   Tuberculosis in children

The concept

Tuberculosis is a serious illness of children, the younger the child, the more serious the illness. The commonest source of infection is an adult in the family or neighbourhood.

Introducing the concept

Ask about the common manifestations of *adult* tuberculosis? Do the people consider it to be a dangerous illness. Do they think it is infectious. What can be done to prevent the spread of infection in the family?

Points to stress

Harmful effects
In children it does not start as in adults with cough and sputum — but the harmful effects can be worse. The common symptoms are:
● loss of weight, lethargy, fever off and on to start with and later becoming persistent, cough and irritability;
● lump on the back in the midline and child later paralysed or unable to walk;
● swelling in the neck;
● pains and swelling of the abdomen and loose stools;
● pain in the hip or knee, causing limp and pain on walking;
● drowsiness and death caused by TB affecting the brain.

It is spread from infected adults to children when they:
● breathe and cough in an overcrowded home with poor ventilation;

- spit on the floor;
- have close contact e.g. sharing a bed.

Prevention
- Persuade adults with a cough which continues, and especially if they have sputum, to get treatment at the clinic.
- Good food, fresh air, ventilation in the house, and sunlight — for all.
- Take the child regularly to the Under-5 Clinic. If the child's weight remains on the 'path to health' there is no need to worry. If weight gain stops, the staff there will help you.
- **Most important:** BCG immunisation. Newborns should have it, but if your child is older he/she can still have it. And a booster dose at 4–5 years old.

Talk 17   Worms

The concept

Intestinal parasites are common. Usually they indicate the extent of environmental pollution. Heavy infections can cause blockage in the gut or loss of blood.

Introducing the concept

Ask whether they have seen worms being passed in the stools of their children: How do they get into the child's gut?

Points to stress

There are different kinds of worm that affect the child in different ways.

Round worm
- **They cause** loss of appetite — loss of weight — they affect growth and occasionally block the intestine.
- **Spread** is from faeces — to food or drinking water — maybe to fingers of people who prepare food.

- **Avoid** by:
- having and using proper latrines;
- washing hands after going to latrine and before eating food;
- washing fruit and vegetables before eating — and boiling water if doubtful;
- keeping food covered to protect from flies.
- **If the child has worms** go to the clinic for treatment.

Hookworm
- Called this name because they 'hook' on to the inside of the gut and so:
- they cause biting pains;
- they suck the blood from the child;
- the child becomes pale and lethargic.
- **Spread** occurs when stools with hookworm eggs are passed on to the ground. The young hookworms come out of the eggs and enter the body through the soles of the feet and make their way to the gut where they fix themselves by the 'hook' to get blood.
- **Avoid** by:
- teaching children to use a proper latrine;
- wearing sandals to protect the feet from the young hookworm.
- **If your child** has biting pains in the belly — and is listless and pale — perhaps it is hookworm. Get some treatment, and avoid it in future.

● CHAPTER 22

Designing and Running a Children's Ward

There are ten factors to be considered.
1 The comfort and care of the occupants are more important than administrative convenience.
2 There tend to be a lot more ill children admitted than the number of cots available.
3 There is usually a shortage of trained and skilled staff. The quality of care depends on the knowledge and devotion of the nursing staff rather than buildings and equipment.
4 The mother's presence and active involvement in the nursing care of the child is vitally important whatever the age of the child.
5 There will be a great variety of medical conditions in one ward; and possibly surgical patients will also be admitted to the same ward.
6 Ages will vary from a few hours, through infancy to childhood.
7 Nutrition is an essential aspect of the care of children, and food should be *specially* prepared for them.
8 It is good to have a place where the mothers can congregate, where staff can teach and demonstrate, and where children, when well enough, can play.
9 Toilets, sluices and washing facilities should be made clean and attractive.
10 The atmosphere or spirit in the ward *can* be one of peace, confidence and hope even though the children are very sick and the work is demanding.

Detailed comments on each of these factors follow.

The comfort and care of the occupants are more important than administrative convenience.

The occupants include not only the children and their parents but also the staff, the ward sister, doctors, staff nurses, students, auxiliaries, cleaners and assistants of every kind. Such *people* are more important to the health of the children than the *building* or type of cots. The patients realise this and they attend a certain hospital in large numbers because they want to be treated by certain people. They avoid another hospital or department in a hospital because 'the doctors are not good or the nurses are not kind!'

In the same way the staff should realise that their primary aim is to care for sick children and comfort their anxious parents. Their primary aim is not the order in the ward, or getting the injections done or filling in the order book correctly. Yet in many hospitals the student nurse is instructed that the duties she has to learn are: the giving of medicines; taking and charting temperatures; being in charge of the milk room; doing the dressings and so on. So she may go around 40 patients 3 times during her shift, doling out tablets and medicines and charting them. She has had no time to get to know the 40 patients as people. The medicine round has become her prime interest. Obviously all these jobs have to be done, and all these techniques have to be learnt. The sole purpose of having the children's ward at all is to heal the patients, viz. the children. And so the children are the most important item in the ward or rather the child-with-mother.

Care should be patient-oriented, not task-orientated

So from the first day in the ward, the ward staff should have responsibility or shared responsibility for a certain number of patients. If there are 6 student nurses and 40 patients then it is possible for them to work in pairs and have special responsibility for 13 patients each. This does not mean rejection of the other patients. Inexperienced staff are not capable of absorbing information and getting to know 40 patients simultaneously. If really interested they could get to know 12 or 13, although 8 would be a better number for the new nurse.

If, for example, there are 2 staff nurses, 4 auxiliaries and 40 patients, then each auxiliary could take a greater interest in an assigned 10 patients. The mothers then feel that they have someone who is especially caring for them, someone who has time for them, someone to report to when the child's condition changes. It is not uncommon in very busy paediatric wards for mothers to take their children home against medical advice! This is often due to the fact that the mother has been worried for days about something and no one has had time to listen to her. When she says she is going, the 'advice' comes, but by then she has made up her mind.

What does this 'responsibility' imply? Ideally it should include all aspects of care for the special patients.

- Getting to know the parents and the family, and establishing good rapport. Obtaining information about the home background.
- Gathering information about the child's progress and needs, the mother's attitude, the ward facilities or lack of them – from her own observations.
- Getting together with all the staff and sharing this information.
- Discussing and planning with all concerned to meet the needs.
- Returning to patient care with a clearer idea of what is going on.
- Assessing with all the staff how the plan is going – at regular staff meetings e.g. weekly or twice weekly.

It also implies a place in the general responsibility for the other patients, the ward and the equipment. For example, with assigned responsibility for a certain number of patients, the cry might be 'It's impossible, everyone would want the medicine trolley at the same time'. Again the staff could sit down and make a plan. It would need *some* reorganisation. In actual fact all patients do *not* get their medicines simultaneously – the trolley goes round one after another – so it's not the trolley that changes but the person giving out the medicine.

Night time

At this time the situation is very different. The staff are much fewer, with 2 or even sometimes 1 nurse in charge of a large ward. She may be expected to complete tasks and treatments far in excess of any day staff. This should be brought to the notice of senior staff and doctors and discussed. It may then be seen that routine duties, special observations and care of new admissions is an overwhelming amount of work in a large ward for 1 or 2 people. Some plan can be made.

There will always be a lot more ill children admitted than the number of available cots.

The aim of the children's ward is to care for those who are too ill to be treated as outpatients. This means that these patients have to be given treatment, whether it is medicine, an injection, an intravenous drip, a nasogastric feed, a dressing and so on. When there are extra children lying on the floor there are literally too many bodies in the area, so the nurses cannot get to the patients to administer the treatments. Or else the number and volume of treatments to be carried out increase so much that they are not given as often as they should be. Nurses become overworked and confused, treatments are done in a hasty and slipshod way, fluids are forgotten, hyperpyrexia is missed, *no one* is treated satisfactorily.

So what can be done?

Long term

● Keep on pressing for prevention, the necessity for immunisations to be available daily and *health education*.

● If preventive action is taken *this* month, then *next* month there will be fewer measles patients admitted. Prevention in the whole community must be organised – it is not sufficient to immunise only those who come to the clinic. All those who do not or cannot should also be reached.

● Overcrowding is the most difficult problem and has defied solution in every type of hospital. This is one area where doctors and ward staff need to assess the situation at least daily. Close liaison between the ward and admission staff, and doctors on emergency duty is essential. It may be useful to have a 'holding' ward in or near the out-patients where day cases may receive treatment like, for example, oral rehydration. After some hours the majority of the children will be able to go home, and return for review the next day.

● Do not order injections when oral medicines are just as good; do not order 8 or 12 hourly injections when daily injections

288

will do. This will cut down the need for admission.

● If in spite of all this there are still too many patients requiring special treatments, then a mother and child hostel may be considered, thus leaving the ward for the more acutely ill. The children from the hostel could get treatment from the out-patients or the 'day' care area depending on the local plan.

There is usually a shortage of trained staff.

Mother's presence is vitally important to the child at the time of sickness and distress. It is important for her too to be able to give *her* love and care. But the mother is also important to the ward staff. Those in charge of the ward could ask themselves 'What is it that I am doing that a staff nurse could do, after I have taught her?'. Then what is the staff nurse doing that the junior nurse could do — when we have taught her? Then down the line to the auxiliaries and last but not least 'What could the mother do that we are doing — after we have taught her?'.

The mothers' presence in the ward makes it look more untidy, they sometimes hold the staff up by talking, they sometimes cause confusion in the toilets and washing rooms. But every nurse in the busy peripheral hospital knows that without the mothers the children would be unhappy and screaming; they would have to be constantly talked to and comforted; they would have to be fed and washed regularly; that every treatment would require an extra person to hold and comfort the child; that the work would never be done. So from this point of view alone, the mothers are a blessing.

It is necessary to be specific in our teaching when delegating to others. To ask for some task to be carried out is not enough. A junior will often walk away after such an order and try and carry it out without really knowing what she is trying to do. So the golden rules are:

● Say what you want done.
● Have it written down so it can be referred to (if dealing with those who can read).
● Show in detail how it is to be done 2 or 3 times.
● Watch the other person doing it a couple of times.
● Leave them alone at it.
● Check a few days later to see how it is going.

Then each person in the ward should really know what jobs they are responsible for – or to put it another way – they should have a **job description**. If no one has yet got one in a ward, then it is good to ask each person to write out their own. If, for example, a cleaner or labourer cannot write, they can say it aloud and someone else can write it down. In this way they are really helped to think about what they are doing every day. Some may realise for the first time that they really aren't doing very much.

There is one attitude that can creep into a ward and that is 'That's not my work so I won't do it'. This is often said by those who do not feel involved in caring for the sick. They only want to get a job done as soon as possible so as to return home to the family and farm. But if they felt needed and important in the ward and they believed they were part of a team sharing the work of healing the sick, then a spirit of cooperation might emerge.

The mothers

If the mothers are to be in the ward they also need to have:
- toilet facilities;
- washing and bathing facilities;
- laundry facilities;
- food – and if they are some distance from home they may want to cook;
- a place to put their 'things' securely;
- a place to sleep.

The ideal situation is to have a mothers' hostel where these facilities are supplied in a simple way. There will have to be *some* rules about the mothers in the ward, otherwise they could be helpful in one way and could obstruct the nurses in another.

From experience one would recommend fathers being involved in discussion about the child's illness and the treatment being carried out. They are more able to influence grandparents and others who give or advise on traditional treatments. Senior wives can also be a problem as are some indigenous doctors. The husband has the authority. In early discharge it is essential for the mother to have support in the community whether urban or rural; and the child's father, or in his absence a senior male member of the family, is an ally.

290

There will be a great variety of medical conditions in one ward.

Patients in *children's hospitals* are grouped *together* to facilitate their care. For example:
● surgical patients in all surgical wards;
● neonate and small infants in a nursery.

But in a children's ward in a small peripheral hospital you may see children with the following conditions being nursed in one ward: measles; whooping cough; poliomyelitis; neonatal tetanus; diarrhoea including cholera; yellow fever; infectious hepatitis; acute purulent meningitis; tuberculosis; lung abscess; discharging wounds.

How should one plan a ward to cater for all these possibilities and avoid cross infection? If one went down the list saying 'Should this condition be isolated − and this?' the answer almost certainly would be 'yes' and one would end up with a corridor with a series of cubicles coming off it.

There are reasons why this type of plan does not work in practice. Mothers will not be happy. They find it a 'cultural shock' to come from the familiarity and cosiness of their houses to be cooped up in a cubicle with hospital cots, electric lights and uniformed personnel. They derive comfort and support from the close proximity of other mothers. Isolation cubicles increase their sense of loneliness and anxiety and they will either come out to mix with others, carrying their sick child with them, or else leave the hospital. Nursing care in cubicles tends to be less rather than more.

In peripheral hospitals in the afternoon and night shifts there may be 2 or *even* only one trained nurse. **It is vital that she is able to observe and know what is happening**. This is more likely when she can *see what is happening*. So that the fewer walls, cubby holes and partitions, the better.

It is hoped that in a few years this particular problem will no longer arise because *all* children will be immunised and vaccinated. But until then one way to solve this particular problem is to have the following organisation.
● Some groups of patients in certain areas i.e. have larger cubicles.

- One or 2 **isolation wards**.
- A few — say 4 or 5 — **isolation cubicles**.
- The **open ward**.

Groups in certain areas (larger cubicles)
- Surgical patients.
- Neonates and small infants.
- Diarrhoea patients.
- Possibly those with severe malnutrition.
- The most critically ill.

Neonates could be in special small cots in an area protected from cold in the wet season.

The word 'diarrhoea' covers a variety of conditions and the majority of patients are not infectious. It is useful to have one area for these children because nurses use gowns when nursing them. The reason for this is that one may not know on admission *which* child is a danger to others and which may be a mild case of cholera. If there are 1 or 2 with obvious cholera, they can be put in an isolation cubicle immediately.

It is very helpful to have *the most* critically ill like, for example, neonatal tetanus, close to the nurses' station. In the daytime, staff may be plentiful but in the night there may be only 1 or 2 staff on duty and it is a great help to have the children near to the nurses' station. Of course the ideal solution is to have an **intensive care unit** and to have the critically ill children away from the general ward, but the above is a suggestion if this is not possible.

Isolation
The questions to be asked are: Is this child likely to transmit his infection to others and *to be a danger* to others? In our practical experience is this condition *actually* transmitted to others in the children's ward? In the case of measles and whooping cough the answer to the above questions is definitely 'yes'. So for the present an **isolation ward** for measles **with its own toilet and washing facilities**, is necessary.

It is often said that the other patients probably meet these measles patients in the out-patients and have already become infected by them. They also may *not* have become infected. When we consider that these other children may have malnutrition, kwashiorkor, severe anaemia, severe broncho-pneumonia or primary tuberculosis *it is wrong* to place these children in close contact with measles and whooping cough. When they succumb to this added infection it will be likely to tip the scales against them and cause a fatality.

Isolation cubicles
About 4 to 6 isolation cubicles are also useful for patients with early acute poliomyelitis, cholera, miliary tuberculosis, measles and whooping cough, and infected wounds. The isolation ward and cubicles should have separate toilet and washing facilities.

Are isolation and intensive care units really possible? Experience has shown that these units allow for better care and are economical in overall staffing and rapid turnover of patients. It is an uphill task to convince the planners since the initial costs seem high. Medical and nursing staff should begin by arranging the wards they have, and then tackle administration for a planned unit. It has been done; success depends on maintaining enthusiasm and demonstrating to the authorities the value of these special areas.

Ages will vary widely. There will have to be a variety of cot sizes. When space is limited it is helpful to have a number − about a fifth − of the cots of infant size. It is easier to nurse an infant and keep him warm in a small cot. A few 'junior' beds are useful for toddlers and the rest can be medium size cots.

Food and nutrition is a vital aspect of caring for sick children in developing countries.

This involves:
● facilities for cooking; and
● a special milk kitchen or diet kitchen for the preparation of special diets for the malnourished.

Children's kitchen
The purpose of this is to supply better food than the child would get either from home or from a general hospital kitchen which would be catering mainly for adults.

An even more important reason why it is valuable to have a children's kitchen near the ward is that demonstration cooking lessons could take place on the verandah. Mothers would then see and taste as well as *hear* about good food.

Milk room
This is essential for the preparation of high energy diets and other fluids so frequently required.

It is essential to have a place where mothers can congregate, where demonstrations and discussions can take place and where children can play.

The second aim of the children's ward is to teach the mothers about their children's condition and how to prevent the illness in future; how to care during convalescence; and also to discuss the care and feeding of healthy children. A great deal of practical education at the one-to-one level can continue throughout the day – at the cotside, while the child is being washed, while meals are being served and so on. But it is also useful to have a place where many mothers can come together and have a talk and exchange views about particular matters.

This could be the same area as the *play* area, which would be of inestimable value.

A really large verandah is a possible place for such activities. The disadvantage of having this 'area' *inside* the building is that sooner or later someone will come along and use it for something else, or else put more beds in it!

Toilets, sluices and washing facilities may be attractive or repellent.

They may be repellent either visually or because of the smell!

It is unattractive, when standing in a ward, to be able to look right down into the toilet area. It is just as easy to plan the toilets so that they are not so obvious.

Anyone who has worked in rural areas knows that water supplies tend to be intermittent, and pumps tend to break down. Therefore it is very important to have plenty of blow-through ventilation, to have an open space between the ward and the toilet area – and to have open windows or open *areas* in the top of the walls.

The atmosphere or spirit in the ward can be one of peace and hope, even though the children are very sick and the work is demanding.

Every children's ward has its own character or 'atmosphere'. This atmosphere can be sensed very quickly. It may be one of hope, of despair, an atmosphere of work done unwillingly or sometimes an atmosphere of apparent resentment to each new mother and child who appears. This happens when the staff feel overworked, they are not sure what they should do, or why they are doing it, and when they see little result for their work.

But when there is a *team spirit* amongst the staff, and support and appreciation from the ward sister and doctor, their morale is high. There *can* be an attitude of hope and even joy when mothers and their children realise that the staff really desire their health and happiness. When the staff consciously realise that their work is to share in the healing of the sick, then the mother and child sense this and the healing process starts.

Later the mother *sees* the child improving and is then more receptive to advice about prevention and immunisation. If she is relaxed then she will express what is on her mind, especially her fears with regard to sickness. In this atmosphere she comes to realise that perhaps what these nurses and doctors are claiming *is* true. Perhaps she *can* prevent sickness by coming to the Children's Clinic. These nurses and doctors seem to know what they are doing, her child has become well.

It is possible to get rid of measles, whooping cough, tetanus, polio and other diseases, as has been done in many countries. The people must *want* prevention. Our part is to show it is possible.

Ten quick basic rules

These are especially useful for newcomers or for doctors or nurses who do occasional duty in the children's ward.

1 **One patient to one bed – or cot.**
  ● Never two in a bed. (If you have too many patients no one will get proper care.)
  ● Also no extra patients on the floor, if you can help it.

2 **Children need to have a relative with them, usually their mother.**
  ● Not two or three family members.
  ● Not another child except in unusual circumstances, for

example if the mother is nursing a baby, and an infected children's ward is not a good place for babies to be brought into.

● If the mother has another child she can:

— leave him at home in the care of someone else;

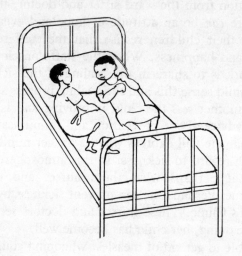

Never two to a bed

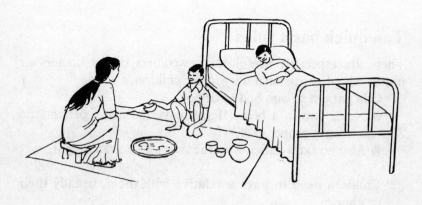

Not too many relatives

– stay at home if she has another small baby and visit when she is able. If she wishes she could leave another responsible relative with the sick child.

3 **Mothers or the relative may eat outside in a special area e.g. an extra large covered verandah, where tables and benches are provided.**

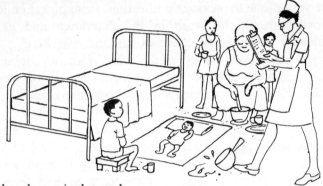

The obstacle race in the ward

Not this!

4 **A store is provided for the mothers to keep their belongings securely.** Do not allow leftover food in the bedside lockers. That will attract cockroaches and rats!
5 **Mothers may sleep by their children at night – but should not lie in the ward in the daytime and so obstruct the nurses.** They may rest on the verandah in the shade.

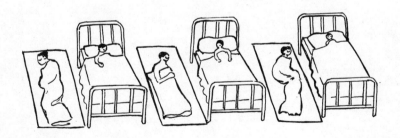

Mothers sleep by the cot side – but not during the day!

6 Children with measles must not be admitted to the general ward but instead be nursed in the measles ward.
7 Children with whooping cough or those on observation for whooping cough must also be admitted to isolation.
8 The critically ill are best placed in the area near the nurses' station where they can be readily observed.
9 Aim at keeping the infants' cubicle for infants only. They are very prone to picking up infections from bigger children.
10 Gowns should be worn in the diarrhoea and cholera cubicles (even when there is no one watching) — and never put charts on the bed. Isolation gowns for nursing children with cholera and diarrhoea are a controversial point. Here are 2 comments from experienced people.

Against They give a false sense of security and are wrongly worn even when clearly marked. Busy doctors rushing from one emergency to another rarely use them. Good hand washing facilities are essential, and so is the care of bed linen and excreta.
For The nurse needs protection — she goes to her lunch, rests her hands (presumably washed) in her lap, is contaminated by her clothing and then eats.

Suggest a plastic gown is worn when attending these patients, and wiped down with Savlon 1% before removal. (A bowl and cloth should be provided just outside the area.) The plastic should be patterned, so that the inside and the outside are clearly recognisable.
So — meet, discuss and make your own decisions on this!

CHAPTER 23

Play

This is often not given enough consideration. We say our aim is to treat not diseases but children i.e. people. A hospital is not a *factory* where cool efficiency is the most desirable attitude. We should be not only efficient but *loving* towards the children and mothers. *Love* is knowing, caring for, respecting and responding to the needs of the other. We do fairly well in the first three, not so well in the last.

A **child's needs** are:
● to feel well, not in pain, not hungry or cold;
● to feel loved, wanted and happy;
● to develop his/her own self through interaction with people, things and life in general.

One vital way the child interacts is by **play**. Play is as important for children as occupation is for adults.
Play:
● gives a sense of well being;
● brings children and adults together to interact with each other;
● when it is creative, helps the child's development and skills.

What can we do to respond to these needs?
● The *very ill children* could be in one area and those who are recovering in another area, away from the perpetual drama and the air of anxiety.
  ● Most of the ill children are in pain or feeling low — try not to increase their suffering by giving unnecessary injections.
  ● Know and respect their need to *feel loved* by wanting the

mothers not only with and near them but also holding them whenever it is possible.

● We should also respect the mothers and not expect them to do nursing duty 24 hours a day – they also need to sleep and eat.
● Lastly, the most neglected item is **the need for play**.
But, the argument is:
– there is no space and no time; and
– this is not the place for play but the place for treatment of disease.

But consider a hospital admission
At first there is great activity, history taking, examinations, treatments and maybe tests.

Then the activity dies down and the child improves slowly.

Then there is renewed activity when the mother and staff are satisfied, instructions are given, belongings collected and the child prepared to go home.

This middle phase is a period of calm when the mother and child *are* receptive and at this time play is helpful.

We must face up to it
Do we only intend to 'cure disease and alleviate pain' or are prevention and health education still on the programme?

If you decide they are, then make facilities for play available
● A place
– It may be a covered area between two buildings – and a pleasant open space as well, if possible.
– Put out mats in the open space with some toys where the mothers and children can sit whilst ward cleaning is going on. Have a swing, a slide or a see-saw for the older children.
● Encouragement by nurses, doctors, students, auxiliaries, so that it is understood that playing is not 'wasting valuable time'.
● Ideally one person or a group of people, maybe nurses or students or volunteers, to supervise play and help with the arrangements daily. They would:
– know the children's games played locally;
– know the dances – a drum is helpful;

– keep an eye on toys such as balls, bricks, blocks, boards with pegs.

The support from doctors, nurses and students as well as their participation in the activity is important. Accusations of time wasting are common in wards as well as play areas. One still finds that senior nurses expect everyone to keep moving. The creation of a relaxed atmosphere is an art, and the good ward sister will appreciate the domestic who stands on her broom chatting to mothers, and the nurse who sits beside the cot as if she had all the time in the world.

The effects of play
● The mothers
– seem to come to life instead of sitting listlessly and brooding by the child's cot;
– relate better to staff and to each other;
– feel more at home;
– learn to provide opportunities for play at home.
● Children
– are delighted;
– realise that clinics and hospitals are no longer fearsome places.
● Staff
– finally realise it doesn't *waste* time but *saves* time because of the cooperation of the mothers and children in other aspects of child care.

CHAPTER 24

Communicating in the Children's Ward

Orientation of a nurse to a children's ward

It is useful for the newcomer, whether it be a nurse, a medical student or a junior doctor unfamiliar with paediatrics, to have an outline giving a bird's eye view of what goes on in the children's ward. The trained staff are usually very busy and patient care tends to take priority over teaching and explaining things to the newcomer. Some hospitals may have clinical tutors but not all.

If there is a written outline of important facts about the care of sick children, then the newcomer can get oriented in an intelligent way. Some new things can be learned each day and checked off on the list as they are seen and experienced.

In medicine and nursing many believe that we learn best by a combination of methods — partly by systematically covering the individual points to be learned, and partly by the day to day work as it crops up in the endless variety of hospital experience.

Orientation outline

The aims of the paediatric ward
● To cure if possible; if not possible, to alleviate pain and discomfort.
● To impart health education to the mother — and convince her of the necessity of follow-up care for consolidating cure.

The place
● The ward — cubicles — isolation facilities.
● Toilets and washing facilities.
● Treatment room.

- Milk room and kitchen.
- Mothers' facilities.

Important facts concerning sick children
- 75% of the children admitted have a *preventable* condition. Malnutrition is common. It undermines health by reducing resistance to infection and contributes to death. Because children are sick, they often refuse fluids and can become dehydrated very rapidly. Maintenance of hydration requires constant vigilance. The mother's presence is of great importance as she gives special care to the child.
- Admission to the children's ward can be a danger to life if the child is exposed to measles and whooping cough there.

Daily ward routine
This should be worked out in each individual ward remembering the necessity for each nurse to have special responsibility for a given number of allotted patients.

Procedures
The junior nurse and the doctor should become knowledgeable and skilled about the following.
- Approaching a child and mother.
- Measuring temperature – counting pulse – apex beat and taking blood pressure.
- Weighing and charting the weights.
- Obtaining a urine specimen.
- Testing urine.
- Tuberculin test.
- Admission routine.
- Bathing.
- Giving medicines.
- Giving injections.
- Oral fluids:
  - special fluids;
  - nasogastric tube feeding;
  - infant feeding chart.

- I.V. fluids: – types;
  - setting up drips;

303

- child's position;
- use and misuse of restrainers;
- follow up;
- charting.
● Blood transfusion.
● Treatment of
- hyperpyrexia;
- hypothermia;
- convulsions.
● Care of eyes;
- ears;
- mouth;
- nose.
● Resuscitation.
● Clinical procedures:
- lumbar puncture;
- pleural tap;
- pleural drainage;
- liver tap;
- paracentesis of the abdomen;
- aspiration;
- tracheostomy;
- exchange transfusion;
- using humidifier.

Care of equipment
● General – same as in other wards.
● Special.

Milk room
● General care and procedures.
● Milk protein diet.
● Electrolyte fluid.
● Lactose-free diet.

Nursing care
● Diarrhoeal diseases.
● Fever – malaria.
● Respiratory infections.
● Measles.

304

- Malnutrition.
- Tetanus.
- Convulsions.
- Meningitis.
- Anaemia.
- Poliomyelitis.
- Skins.
- Accidents.
- Neonates:
  - prematurity;
  - inability to suckle at the breast;
  - spasms;
  - jaundice;
  - distended abdomen;
  - 'not doing well';
  - sticky eyes;
  - skin infections.

Diet instruction
- Preparing special diets for babies and children.

Health education
- Understanding and teaching about under-5 weight charts.
- Immunisation and vaccination. Malaria prophylaxis.
- Talks on the following topics.
  - Antenatal care.
  - Delivery.
  - Newborns.
  - Under-5 weight chart.
  - Under-5 Clinic.
  - Circumcision.
  - Purges and enemas.
  - Feeding.
  - Immunisation.
  - Malaria prophylaxis.
  - Crying too much.
  - Water.
  - Dangers of feeding bottles.
  - Worms.
  - Latrines.

- The compound.
- The school child's health.
- Rehydration.
- Prevention of: diarrhoea; cholera; tetanus; whooping cough; malaria; TB; and measles.
- Responsible parenthood and family planning.

Planning to cover the material in title outline

This is an individual matter for the ward staff in each hospital. The content of training also depends on the length of time each nurse will spend in the children's ward. One thing is essential: **a specific person should teach specific items on specific days** or else the days will slip by and little is accomplished.

For example

Day 1	General introduction to the ward and walk around the ward.
	● Talk on **cross infection**. See isolation areas, pages 292–3. Importance of separating measles and whooping cough patients from the others.
	● Talk on **cleanliness**. See toilets – washing areas – sluices, page 294.
	● Talk about **mothers staying** with their children. Where mothers sleep, wash, eat and store their things.
	● Importance of good food and **nutrition**. See where children's food is cooked, page 293. See milk kitchen, page 294.
	● Importance of **safety**. Safe cots: narrow space between bars, no gaps between bottom rail and base. Tutor demonstrates how to take and chart temperature – pulse and apex beat.
	● Stress the importance of learning some new things every day and ticking off the items as they are understood and experienced.

	● The facts to be taught are arranged in groups and headed DAY 1, DAY 2 etc. as a rough guide.
	(The following has been the practice at one small hospital, and it is realised that every hospital has its own somewhat different routines.)
Day 2	● **Re-emphasise nutrition**. Demonstrate weighing scales and let each nurse practise under supervision.
	● Fill in weight charts as exercise. Do exercise in judging growth from the weight graph. Fill in the patient's own chart.
	● **Urine specimens** – How to *obtain* and how to test.
	● **Tuberculin test.**
	● **Admission of patient**.
Day 3	**Infant feeding charts.**
	● **Care of children on I.V. fluids.**
	● **Filling in I.V. fluid charts.**
Day 4	● Immunisation – vaccination – malaria prophylaxis
Day 5 *Day 6*	● **Care of equipment.**
	– Same as in adults' wards – beds (cots) lockers, screens and trolleys.
	– Weighing scales,
	– Suction apparatus.
	– Croupaire.
	– Importance of immediate repair.
Day 7	● **Awareness of the patient's condition and progress.**
	● **How to report this to senior staff and on doctors' rounds.**
Day 8 and *Day 9*	● **Emergency treatments.**
	– Collapse – resuscitation.
	– Hyperpyrexia.
	– Convulsions.

	– Hypothermia.
	– Dehydration.

Day 10 and *Day 14*	● **Procedures.**
	– Nasogastric tube – how to pass and how to feed.
	– Oral suction.
	– Oral toilet.
	– Type of care for measles patients.
	– Use and misuse of restrainers if the child is receiving I.V. fluids or feeds through the nasogastric tube.
	– Preparation for – I.V. infusions;
	      – lumbar puncture;
	      – pleural tap.
	– Rectal swab for cholera.
	– The cleaning of ears.
	– Treatment of scabies.
	– Blood transfusion.

Day 15 *Day 16*	**Surgical routines.**

Throughout the stay in the children's ward the following must be taught:
● experience in caring for the various conditions;
● experience in teaching prevention and health education;
● experience in the milk room.

All the trained core staff on the ward should be teachers – passing on their skills and experience to the newcomers.

Where there is no clinical tutor or instructor, the sister in charge of the ward may assign the responsibility of teaching to a reliable staff nurse. The ward sister or charge nurse is still the most valuable teacher. There is a tendency nowadays to leave teaching to tutors which is detrimental to good ward practice, especially in the case of children. New doctors and medical assistants as well as nurses benefit most from the experience of a ward sister.

Ward rounds

This is an important time for communication between the staff, when observations are exchanged and decisions taken regarding the management and care of the patient. It is important that time is not wasted in looking for records and reports and all requirements are anticipated.
● On the trolley there should be:
– diagnostic set, spatulas, kidney dish;
– continuation sheets, laboratory forms and X-ray forms;
– percussion hammer – B.P. apparatus;
– a note book for taking down notes regarding the management of patients.
● Always carry a note book to write down personal notes and to remind you of any observations which you may wish to report.
● A child will cry if approached quickly and undressed in a great hurry. So approach quietly, take the cot side down gently, and only prepare for examination if requested.
● Be ready to report the condition of the patient since the last ward rounds if the patient is your responsibility. Consult your notes to help you to do this.
● Learn how to hold a child to have:
– ears examined, lying and sitting;
– throat examined, lying and sitting.
● Learn how to assemble the auriscope.

Matron's round

Unfortunately the formal round from matron's office still continues as a tradition, with everyone trying to look very business-like and efficient. Matrons should meander round the ward alone, and talk to mothers and the nurse caring for a particular child. It is a useful method of assessing the nurse's knowledge without her being aware of being tested and the nurse gives a more spontaneous response. With patient-oriented care, the nurse always gives the report to doctor, sister, matron, and the mother. Doctors as well as senior nurses need to be persuaded of the value of this.

It is useful to bear in mind that the doctor is with each

patient for a few minutes only each day (sometimes less). The nurse is near the patients most of the time and has a good insight into their progress, yet sometimes nurses feel that their observations do not matter and keep silent at ward rounds. Often the doctor is at a loss to know what to do next for a patient, and the nurse has the valuable information which would help to make a decision. It is better to speak about the fluid chart, the weight curve or anything else which may contribute to decision making than to keep silent. The nurses' observations do have a very important purpose.

When giving a report on your patients on ward rounds

You will not have an intimate knowledge of your patients' condition unless you are closely involved in their care and *observe* them. But it does help to know what to look for. Think first about the presenting complaint and the probable diagnosis. Find out about the progress of the presenting complaint and relevant facts about the diagnosis.

If diarrhoea

● Stools   How many during the last 24 hours (not since morning). Describe − Type (normal − formed − loose − water − colour) − with mucus − with blood − foul smelling − with undigested matter.
● Vomiting also   How many in 24 hours? What it looked like? Was it vomiting only:
− after coughing?
− after medicine?
− after feeding?

Tell parents to *show* you all stools and vomits and discuss with them.
● Drinking   Is the child drinking? Enough? Has the mother been encouraging this? Needs nasogastric drip?
● If on I.V.
What was intake during 24 hours? − output in 24 hours? What is the state of hydration now?

310

If malnutrition

● Sucking – Appetite (good, fair, very poor).
  Whether child takes enough orally or needs intragastric feeding. What was the intake in 24 hours, say 8 a.m. yesterday – 8 a.m. today?
● Any vomiting?
● What *food* was he able to retain in the last 24 hours?
● Weight? Gaining? Losing?
● Oedema?
● Personality – Happy? Unhappy? Any smile yet?
● Mother – Caring? – Intelligent? – Understands the instructions about diet? Home conditions? – What you have learned from the mother?
● Share mother's joy when the child begins to improve.

If high fever

● Temperature – and temperature chart. On aspirin?
● Is the child drinking enough?
● Is the cause known or is it an undiagnosed fever?
● What treatment? Tepid sponge – or fan. What response?

If convulsions

● How many during the last 24 hours?
  Report on time started and finished.
● What part of body affected?
● What treatment? – And what response to treatment?
● Has the child had other convulsions before? – How many?
● What sedation has the child had?
● Fever – subsiding? Is the cause known?
● Was a lumbar puncture done? When? Results?

If tetanus

● Spasms – How severe and how often? – Show spasm chart.
● If collapsed during last 24 hours – was it during spasm? (indicating need for more sedation) or was it when baby was quiet and limp? (indicating that less sedation is required).

- Tone — Is baby hypertonic? — or perhaps limp (and over-sedated)?
- Apex beat — if unusually high e.g. 160 this may be a serious sign — so report.
- *Later* — has sucking reflex returned?
  Is weight maintained even when nasogastric feeding stopped?
- Has baby had BCG? It is a good time to do it now.
  Remember to arrange tetanus immunisation.

If measles

Acute phase
- Temperature.
- Respirations — Rate — Is the child in respiratory distress?
- Fluid intake — Has the child drunk enough in the last 24 hours? Does he need N.G. tube now?
- Is the mouth sore? Look at each eye every day.
- Stools? How many?
- Any special point e.g. Stridor or very sore eyes?
- Mother's beliefs re measles — Does she think child is improving?

After acute phase
- State of nutrition — Weight — Improving? — Is the child on high energy diet? — If so, is he taking enough? — Or does he need nasogastric drip? — Is he eating other foods? If so, which foods? — Is the weight going up or down? Show weight chart.
- Anaemia — Measles masks anaemia — Was routine haemoglobin done? If low — act.
- Secondary infection — If present — is it responding to treatment?
- Education — Does this mother realise measles is preventable — and will she get her next child or other children immunised? Arrange other immunisations for patient when better and report on this.

● CHAPTER 25

Procedures and Charting

Approaching a child and mother

● Remember the usual courtesy when coming to the mother and child in the ward − greet her − and then her presence is acknowledged and her feeling of strangeness and loneliness is less.

● The child who is so used to being carried may be in the cot when you come. Move quietly and slowly so as not to frighten the child. Put the cot sides up or down gently and quietly − do not frighten the child by its jerky noise.

● Take the opportunity to explain to the mother that the cot sides are for the child's protection.

As a rule the mother may hold the child, and this is good for both of them. But the mother has also to be considered − she cannot hold the child all day − she has to eat, wash and sleep. So when she is out for short periods the cot sides keep the smaller child safe.

● Cots are made rather high to make it easier for the staff to nurse the child. If a child falls out, it is quite a distance − therefore put cot sides up and teach the mothers to do it. If you notice the cot sides down, and no one near the child, put them up *even if you were not the one who put them down.*

● Get to know the child's name, and call him by name. One often hears 'Have you given cot 27 his injection?'. Treat all children as people.

Admission of a patient to the children's ward

● **On arrival** If any **urgent tests** or **treatments** have been ordered − attend to these immediately.

- If 2 or 3 patients come in together, **assess** the one who is most sick and **attend to him first.**
- Find out **which cot** or **bed** the newly admitted child will be going to, so it can be prepared.
  Remember
- Measles patients go to the measles ward — and should go immediately, even for admission routine.
- Whooping cough patients should go to isolation room immediately, even for admission routine.

Critically ill patients and all tetanus patients should always be in the area near the nurses' station. Other infants should be in the infants' cubicle. Even though noise and bright light have been reported as precipitating spasms in neonatal tetanus, in practice it is not so if the patient is well sedated. It is touch, movement or the passage of cold fluids down the nasogastric tube which cause spasms in neonatal tetanus.

- Take all particulars and **fill in front of chart.**
- **Weigh and chart.**
- Check that all under 5's have **the Road to Health Chart.** If the family has been issued such a chart and it has not been brought, send a relative to get the chart.
- **Bath** (unless obviously very clean).
  If seriously ill, give a **bed bath,** always with the mother assisting.
- **Heaf test** unless
- has had BCG;
- has had recent Heaf test done;
- is known to have tuberculosis;
- has had measles in last 4 weeks;
- is neonate.
- **Collect urine specimen.**
- **Mother's orientation.** During all this time you can be talking to the mother in a friendly way. Remember she is *worried* because her child is sick, and unsure because she is in a strange place. She sees activities which are culturally strange. People are dressed up in strange uniforms and white coats and wear strange caps on their heads. You can help her to become more confident.

Show mother:
− bathroom and toilet;
− where she may eat on the verandah;
− where her store is.
Introduce her to the other mothers from same village.

If the child has **measles** or is in **isolation**, explain to her why this is. Ask her to leave the child in bed and not to carry the child about with her when she goes out of the ward. Tell her in a few days the child will be out of isolation and able to mix freely with the others. If the mother goes out for a time, allow a domestic or auxiliary to remain with the child if possible.

Temperature, pulse, respiration and blood pressure

Temperature

● Usually taken rectally in infants and children up to 2 years.
● Age 2−10 − axillary.
● Age 10 onwards − orally.

Rectally
Use round bulb thermometers − not a long narrow elongated one. Lubricate and insert very gently into the rectum, remembering that the rectum passes **backward**, not directly upwards.

Orally
Be sure you have a cooperative child.

Pulse

● If the radial pulse cannot be felt, try the femoral.

Apex beat

This is difficult to count when you are not used to it. Practice on children who are not so sick − later try with smaller infants. Ask a senior person to check you until you are competent.

When you are experienced, measuring the rate of the apex beat accurately is of great help in assessing a very ill infant or child.

Respiration

● Always count. It is of great value in diagnosis.

Charting

A graph type of chart is always more valuable than those in which numbers are written.

The purpose of taking these readings and writing them down is because they are *important* in monitoring the progress of a very ill infant. They are messages to us, telling us how the child is doing. This is why they are called *vital signs*.

The graph is important because it can be seen at a glance if there is a certain *trend*. For example, pulse and temperature may both be going up or down.

Or there may be a certain *pattern* − for example the temperature rising every 48 hours. This would not be noticed if the temperatures were recorded as numbers in a column.

Charting of temperature
● Usually temperature is charted morning and evening on the front of the chart. This gives a general pattern.
● For certain reasons, a 4-hourly temperature is charted on a 4-hourly chart: e.g.
− in hyperpyrexia;
− in those running a persistent temperature;
− in premature babies and sick neonates.
● An hourly or even half-hourly temperature recording may be requested − e.g. in hyperpyrexia or hypothermia. In this case it is useful to have a chart recording temperature down to 35°C.

Charting of pulse
Usually taken and recorded at the same time as temperature.
Remember − always be honest − if you cannot feel or count the pulse, do not put down a false number. But tell a more senior person.

316

As children's pulse rates vary widely — maybe 50–200 — cater for this if you are designing a new chart.

Charting of apex beat
Only experienced nurses should take responsibility for taking and charting this.

Blood pressure

Three sizes of cuffs are manufactured:
● adult size;
● child size;
● baby size.

Always use the appropriate size. The cuff should be sufficiently large to extend from the axilla to the antecubital fossa. If too-small a cuff is used, the reading will be false.

Charting
Chart the blood pressure readings on the front of the child's chart if it is measured only once or twice daily. If taken more often, use a special B/P chart.

It is essential to remember normal readings for age, as shown in Table 25.1.

Table 25.1

Age (years)	Average (mean)	
	Systolic	Diastolic
0–2	95	55
3–6	100	65
7–10	105	70
11–15	115	70

But there is a variation, within normal limits, depending on what the child is doing or has been doing recently, e.g. higher if crying or playing actively.

Weighing

Why is it essential to weigh children regularly?
● Because it gives information which we can *measure* concerning the nutritional state. Therefore there is also a measure of improvement or the opposite when the *trend* is observed after several weights are charted at intervals. In oedematous patients it may also give a measure of the amount of oedema fluid. **The nutritional state** is one of the most vital factors in the child's state of health. It is known that those who are poorly nourished become much more seriously ill when suffering from any infection, and are more likely to die. If we are trying to *improve* the state of nutrition we want a way of checking to see if we are succeeding or not.
● It is necessary to know the child's weight so as to work out the drug dosage. Many drugs are dangerous if given in *overdose*, e.g. chloroquine by injection.

All purpose scales
Spring balance hanging from a bar. For use in rural and mobile clinics. This balance is sturdy, accurate and cheap. It is recommended.
● Except for *spring* type weighing scales:
− balance the scales on the beam *before* weighing the child;
− in beam type − always return markers to zero after use.

Charting weights

Weights may be recorded:
● on out-patient card;
● on under-5 card in graph form;
● on admission form on in-patient chart.

Certain patients also have special weight charts e.g. neonates, malnourished children, and children with oedema as in heart disease.

Reporting about weights
It is important to draw the attention of senior colleagues and

318

doctors when the child fails to gain weight or loses weight *so action* can follow.

Under-5 weight charts
Every child must have one.
● Fill in name, family history, numbers, etc.
● Turn the card over and put month and year of birth in first space below graphs on left, e.g. OCT. 87.
● Write in month and year of birth at left lower corner of the graph for each year, e.g. OCT. 88.
● Fill in the months up till current month.
● Chart weight.
● Write reason for special care at top left hand corner, e.g. orphan, premature, twin, 8th child.
● Write any present illness vertically alongside present weight, e.g. measles, diarrhoea, TB.
● Fill in immunisations and vaccinations already given.
● When antimalarial is given, put a ring around the month in which it is given, e.g. DEC. 87

Interpreting the under-5 weight chart
The *slope* of the weight curve is the crucial factor, not the position of a solitary weight recording, so:
– *regular* attendance at clinic, and
– immediate charting of the weight on the graph are important.

The lower line represents the average weight of children growing slowly and the upper line the average weight of children whose growth is adequate. (These lines happen to be equivalent to the 3rd centile for girls and 50th centile for boys in Western Europe.)

The *objective* is to detect faltering of growth early, and intervene immediately if the slope of the growth curve shows a downward trend.

In-patient weight charts
These resemble temperature charts in that there is a space for each day. So someone looking at the chart considers daily weight gain or loss.
● A common mistake is to mark in the weight recording in the

next empty column after the previous one − there may have been a 3 day gap! Avoid this by:
- always filling in *dates* first when you start the chart;
- noting the column for the particular day before making the record.
● Another vital point. These charts are for a *purpose*, yet it does happen that a child is weighed, has lost perhaps 1 kg (2 lbs) in 2 days. It is faithfully charted *but no action is taken*! In case of large fluctuations in weight, re-weigh after checking the accuracy of the machine, especially if it is a beam balance type of weighing scale. If the fluctuation in weight is confirmed, report to a more senior person. This person then has to consider 'why this child has lost weight' and start investigating.

Intravenous infusion

Site of infusion

The aim is to start the I.V. drip in a site where it is most likely to *remain*. It is very traumatic to a child to set up I.V. drips in areas where the fluid nearly always infiltrates − e.g. in front of the elbow.

Needles can be strapped in a stable way:
● in the hand, forearm or foot;
● in the scalp in infants − although avoid scalp vein if any other vein is available.

Have the child restrained well *before* putting the needle in, otherwise it may come out.

Strap diagonally leaving
best vein exposed in the angle

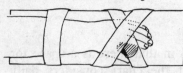 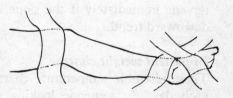

Pad under hand

Restraining the hand   *Restraining the leg*

Intake and output

Fluid charts should be kept down to a minimum, but if a child is to have one, it must be accurately recorded and totalled every 24 hours.

If the child is on fluids by mouth, remind the mother not to drink from the child's drinking-water container. It is wise to consult her about the child's fluid intake before filling in the chart.

Feeding chart

- Chart in mls.
- Write **feed prescribed** once for each day. Not only the *name* of the milk or other preparation but the amount, and also the amount of water, fruit juices and other fluids ingested.
- **Amount taken** in the next column should be filled in when it is ingested *by the child*, not by the mother.
- If the child has malnutrition, always chart the **food taken**.
- **Remark column** can be used to comment on appetite, food, urine, vomit or stool.

Note Observation at meal times is important. Nurses should know and be able to report accurately on the food taken either willingly or with persuasion.

Daily fluid chart

Some charts are designed for use when there is a scale on the infusion bottle. The scale may be on a piece of paper gummed to the bottle.

- Under **remarks** chart the *type* of fluid and the rate of administration e.g. on the first line write:
  Hartmann's 50 ml/hour.
- If there is no hourly scale on the bottle, work out the amount of fluid required, say in 4 hours − then under **remarks** chart:
  Hartmann's 200 ml by noon.
- Check infusion hourly and adjust rate as necessary. As a rule of thumb, a rate of 15 drops per minute equals 1 ml.
- Special attachments are available which allow a small amount

of fluid to be measured and dispensed but these add to the costs of the infusion set.
- The whole chart is valueless unless:
- oral fluids — and output are also charted;
- daily totals are calculated.
- Those who have been managing the infusion for the previous 8 hours, i.e. those on night duty, should do the totals.

Collecting specimens

Urine specimens

Requirements
- For ward examination — clean container.
- For culture — sterile container.

Cooperative older children
- No problem — same as adults.
Uncooperative smaller children
- Plastic bags are ideal, but few hospitals have them at present. When applied, child has to be watched or else he will pull it off.
- If no plastic bag available, a test-tube may be used. A small test-tube is best.

Catheterisation   should be avoided if at all possible on account of the danger of introducing infection.

Suprapubic tap   may be done by a physician if it is very necessary to get a sample of urine for culture, especially in an infant.

Method — The suprapubic area is cleaned, and using a sterile syringe and needle, the bladder area is aspirated. This is a safe procedure when sterile precautions are taken.

Stool specimen

Be quite sure what you are collecting the specimen for, so that it may be collected correctly, and the laboratory request form be filled in properly.

A sterile container is necessary if culture is required.

Testing for cholera
A rectal swab is usually taken and placed directly into alkaline peptone water.

Testing for amoebae in acute diarrhoea
The collected stool should be transferred to the laboratory as soon as it is passed, for immediate examination before the trophozoites die. This happens in less than an hour.

Testing for pathogenic E. coli in infants
Specifically ask for identification of pathogenic *E. coli* – then special tests will be done.

Testing for lactose intolerance
It is necessary to place a piece of plastic inside the nappy to collect the liquid stool so as to avoid absorption into the nappy. The sugar to be tested for is dissolved in the watery part of the stool, and if it is all absorbed into the nappy the test would be inconclusive.

Treatments

A note on giving medicines

Children often do not object to the taste of a medicine but become terrified and struggle because they are suddenly held tight and approached by a nurse with the medicine.

- If possible let the mother give it – but *stay* and *watch* that it is administered.
- If she cannot do it, then help her, but remain calm and quiet, not violent.
- If it really tastes unpleasant, give a drink or something else to take the taste away – then there will be less resistance at the next dose.

When giving injections

Again approach child gently and get the mother's cooperation. Talk to the child before, during and after the injection so that the child can see you are not meaning to *attack* him.

Give the injection as usual in the upper outer quadrant of the gluteal region but remember that however thin a child may be, *never* give the injection in the centre of the buttock because of the danger of causing injury to the sciatic nerve. Make sure that the needle and the syringe have been properly sterilised. **Never try to 'disinfect' a needle by rubbing it with a swab soaked in methylated spirit.**

After giving the injection, hold a swab over the area for a minute or two. Mothers love to rub the area with their hands, but this should be discouraged because of the danger of introducing infection this way.

Routine eye care in measles

Using a swab moistened with plain water or saline, remove any pus from the eyelids, working from the inner canthus outwards. Have a good look at the cornea every day, preferably without manually forcing the lids open − but it may be necessary.

Give Vitamin A in oil orally 200,000 i.u. once as a single dose. Measles causes a 'leak' of the vitamin from the body into the urine, and in communities where xerophthalmia is common it can precipitate an acute deficiency.

The nurse should be the one to notice significant changes, e.g. increasing inflammation, ulceration or severe photophobia.

Then gently pull down the lower lid and insert drops or ointment as prescribed. Report to senior staff if in doubt. Further treatment may be necessary to prevent blindness.

Cleaning discharging ears

Do only when there is a purulent discharge and you have *been shown* how to do it *and are supervised*. Incorrect or careless technique may cause unnecessary pain, abrasion of the meatus, or even perforation of the ear drum. Yet when you are shown carefully how to do it, you may soon acquire the necessary skill.

A common mistake is to use a probe covered thickly with cotton wool. A special metal probe for ears should be used with the minimum amount of cotton wool to cover it. In this way it does not have to be forced down the meatus, causing pain.

Always be gentle. You will nearly always get the child's cooperation. Never force the swab into the ear.

This is the time to remember the possibility of hearing loss. It is often missed and the children are regarded as 'retarded'.

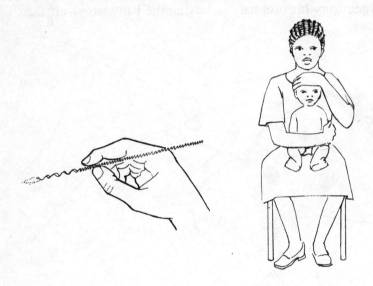

The wire wool carrier

Restraining the hands and steadying the head

Oral toilet in a small child

This can be difficult when children are frightened. But if the child is sitting on the mother's lap, with his back to the mother, he feels more secure. She holds the child's forehead close to her with one hand and holds the child's arms crossed over his chest with her other hand.

The nurse *sits* opposite the child, and holds the lips open gently with the fingers of the left hand. The rest of the procedure is as usual.

Suctioning the nasopharynx

- **Size of tube**   For neonates and small infants use 15 F.G.
- Hold the baby's face with the left hand so that the mouth opens. Insert tube, *without suctioning*, as far as you wish to go. Then apply suction while slowly withdrawing.
- Pause for some seconds to allow the infant to take a breath and to clean out the suction tube. Then repeat the procedure. If you keep applying suction continuously, the infant is unable to breathe, and you are also removing all the air and oxygen from his oropharynx leaving the baby worse off than before.

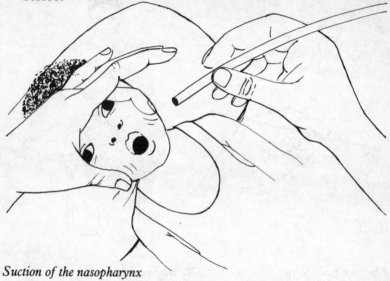

Suction of the nasopharynx

Nasogastric feeding

Passing the nasogastric tube

Requirements
A tray containing:
- N.G. tube in a container (6 F.G. for infants, 8 F.G. for toddlers); (The size of the tube should approximate the size of the little finger of the child.)
- aspiration syringe in a container;

● strapping and scissors;
● restrainers, if necessary, for an older child.

Note A tube made of synthetic material (plastic, polythene or nylon) is better than a red-rubber one, which causes irritation of the mucous membrane. A red-rubber tube may not be left *in situ* in an infant. A synthetic tube may be left *in situ* for up to 7 days but should then be withdrawn, and another tube passed through the other nostril.

Nasal route procedure
● Infants should be lying flat. This is to steady the head, and also to prevent kinking of the pharynx and oesophagus as an infant's head tends to fall forwards.
● Ask the mother to hold the child's hands. If no mother or relative is available another member of staff should help. Only use restrainers if there is no person to help you.
● Measure the distance from the ear to the nose and onto the stomach, and mark the tube at this point.
● Water only is used as a lubricant. Make sure that it does not trickle into the trachea as this could be harmful.
● Control the baby's head and face with the left hand, and with the right hand insert the tube through the nose up to the mark.
● Watch for cyanosis or coughing during the procedure, and if any occurs, withdraw the tube immediately and start again. It may have gone the wrong way!
● Aspirate for stomach contents. Sometimes none comes up, in which case place the end of the tube in a bowl of water. If regular, intermittent or persistent bubbling occurs − the tube is in the respiratory passages − withdraw immediately. Start again.
● When the tube is in the stomach, strap the end to the baby's cheek, and mark the date on the strapping with biro − e.g. 7.3.85.

Possible difficulties
● **Nasal oedema**. If a baby has been on tube feeding for some time, it may be difficult to pass a tube nasally because of oedema. Insert 2 drops of $\frac{1}{2}$% Ephedrine solution in water

into each nostril. Wait for 15 minutes after which oedema may be reduced, and try again.
- **Tetanus spasms**. If there is difficulty in passing a nasogastric tube because of tetanus spasms, do not persist. Sedate the baby well with paraldehyde. Sedation is usually the deepest 20–30 minutes after the injection is given, so commence inserting the nasal tube after 25 minutes.

Oral route procedure
The oral route is used when the nasogastric route is not possible, or when red-rubber tubes are the only ones available. The procedure is the same as for the nasal route except you should insert tube fairly rapidly through mouth into the oesophagus. If you are slow and hesitant, the pharyngeal reflex may occur and cause vomiting.

Giving the feed
- Always start by injecting 3 ml of water slowly down the tube first. Watch for any signs of cyanosis or coughing which would indicate the tube was in the wrong passage. If this occurs, withdraw and start again.
- When you are satisfied the tube is in the stomach:
- if the feed is to be given by a slow drip, run the feed through the tubing and attach the tube to the drip set and bottle containing the feed;
- if the feed is to be given intermittently, connect the barrel of a 20 ml syringe to the tube, and use it as a funnel. Pour the milk into the barrel without using the plunger.
- Allow at least 15 minutes for the feed to go down slowly – the time a child takes to breast feed. If you feed too fast, the baby will vomit.
- Syringe 3 ml of water through the tube after the feed to clean the tube and to avoid milk curdling and blocking it.

Withdrawing the tube
The tube should be pinched while it is being withdrawn, so that any fluid within the tube may not trickle into the pharynx and trachea. It is withdrawn by a slow continuous movement and not too rapidly.

Postural drainage

Description

If you have a pot of water and you want to empty it, you have to tilt it, until the fluid comes out. **This is the principle of postural drainage.** Naturally, the fluid cannot drain as long as the pot remains upright.

A pot of water

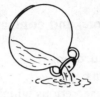

Tilting the pot for emptying

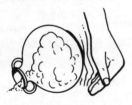

Tapping the pot to help the flow

If the fluid was very thick, you could tap the pot with your hand to help the fluid to come out. **This is clapping.**

A child with infection of the lungs may have secretions in the sponge-like lungs – and either the secretions are:
● so thick;
● or the child is too weak;
● or there is so much (as in lung abscess) that the child cannot cough them out.

So we tilt the child as we tilted the pot, until the secretions drain out and this can be aided by *clapping*.

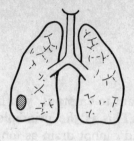

Abscess in the lung

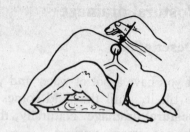

Tilting the child

Indications and contraindications

Postural drainage
Indications
— Excess secretions which the child has difficulty in clearing.

Contraindications
— Children who cannot tolerate the head down position, and some very ill children. Lying flat, or lying on the side may give *some* drainage.

Clapping
Indications
— Thick secretions — from any cause. Lung abscess.

Contraindications
— Tuberculosis — acute infections, empyema, pneumothorax, fractured ribs.

Clapping

This can be learnt with a little practice.

Wrong position   This hurts the patient. Try it on yourself and your colleagues.

Stiff wrist but *cup* your hand and keep it cupped, while your wrist is loose and the movement is *from* the wrist. Try this on

330

your own thigh and on each other and it is not painful. Also, it makes a special sound which you will come to know.

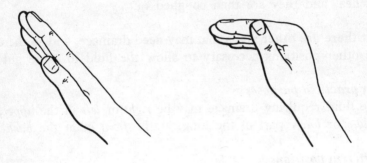

Clapping — wrong position   *Clapping — correct position*

When you do it this way, the child does not mind; if you do it with the stiff wrist and straight hand, the child cries with pain.

The position for postural drainage

● *Why* different positions?
● Because the lungs have different compartments or lobes.

Take a child's X-ray
A view from the front (the usual view). There is a collection of fluid on the *right* at the *base*. The collection is at the *back*. So it is on the *right* at the *base* at the *back*.

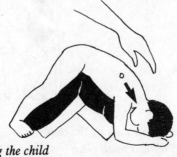

One way of tilting the child

To get the fluid (or pus) out:
● tilt the child for 20 minutes 4 times a day;
● clap over the area for 1–5 minutes during this time.

The thick secretions or pus pass along the bronchus to the trachea, and they are then coughed out.

But there are other areas that may need drainage, and so there are other positions necessary to allow the fluid to come out.

For practical purposes
The fluid requiring drainage may be *right* or *left* in the *upper*, *middle* or *lower* part of the lung, at the *front* or at the *back*.

Different positions
An arrow indicates area to be *clapped* if this is to be done.

Upper lobes
At apex of lobe *or* for the back or posterior part.

Child sitting on a small chair held by mother for the front or anterior part.

Remember, if secretions are on *one* side, put this side *uppermost* to obtain drainage.

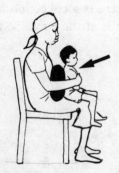 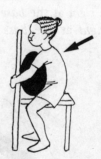

Clapping at the front — mother holding the child
Clapping at the back — using a small chair

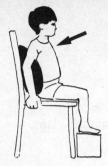
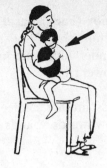

Clapping at the front — using a small chair
Clapping at the back — mother holding the child

Middle lobe (on right) Lingula (on left)
- Lie the patient on his side flat.
- Raise the head side of the bed by 30−35 cm. (12−14 inches).
- Place a pillow from behind to extend from the shoulder to the hips.
- Roll the patient slightly back on the pillow.
- Clap over nipple area.

Lower lobes
For anterior basal area
- Lie the patient on his back.
- Place a pillow under hips and knees.
- Clap at lower ribs.

For lateral basal area
- Lie the patient on right side if draining left lung.

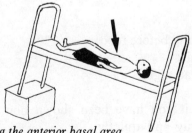

Draining and clapping the anterior basal area

- Lie on left side if draining right lung.
- Place a pillow under hips.
- Clap at lower ribs.

For posterior (back) basal area

● Lie on stomach.
● Pillow under hips and knees.
● Clap at lower ribs,
  or
● Lie across mother's knee.
● Head downwards, hands on floor, mother claps.

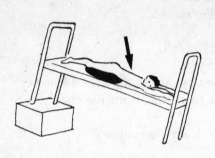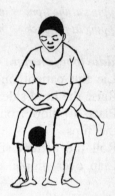

Draining and clapping the posterior basal area
Mother holding and clapping

How often, how long and when

Time

● Postural drainage — 10–20 minutes 4 times a day.
● Clapping — 1–5 minutes of this time, 4 times a day

● Best
— early morning before food;
— before meals;
— last thing at night.

● Only clap if you have been shown how to do it.
● Do it calmly and quietly.
● Start with a short period if the child is fearful, and then increase.
● Keep a chart and write down the number of times it was done and the results, i.e. if fluid came up — its appearance.

334

● CHAPTER 26

Care of Equipment

The need for 'care'

This really includes the care of *all* things because all *things* need caring for. How often we go into a ward and find a light not working. 'For how long?' 'For so long − it happened when I was not on duty!'

It is no good saying 'I reported it' and leaving it at that if nothing happens. Something must be wrong if no action is taken. Is it the method of reporting? Is there no plan of action?

The staff of each ward need to sit down and make their own plan for the *care* of their equipment and for the *procedure* for obtaining new equipment.

An outline of a plan

Basic equipment

Cots
● Dust daily with a damp and dry duster.
● Check bedclothes and mattress. If torn, report to sister so they can be mended.
● Carbolise cot after each patient leaves.
● Clean wheels on cots and trolleys on Saturdays.

Trolleys
● Wash daily.
● Check trolley wheels on Saturdays.
● See that they are oiled periodically.

Dripstands
● Daily dusting with wet and dry dusters.

Weighing scales
● Daily dusting by nurse responsible.

Screens
● Damp dusting daily. Clean wheels on Saturdays.

Wall fan
● One nurse to be responsible.
● Switch off and remove plug when not needed.

Splints
● Nurse removing the splint should remove strapping marks.
● Wash and dry the splint and return to cupboard.

Ear speculae
● Do not boil or autoclave if there are any plastic parts.
● Wash in soap and water then disinfect in Savlon 1% for 1 hour. Then wash, dry and put away.

If there is a rapid turnover of speculae, as for example in the Outpatients, wash in soap and water to remove wax and debris, then sterilise by immersing in Savlon 1–30 in spirit for 3 minutes, Rinse, dry and replace.

As spirit evaporates rapidly, the solution should be kept tightly covered at all times.

As Savlon rusts metals quickly, the speculae should not be left in it any longer than is necessary.

Resuscitation equipment
● Check daily. A senior nurse should be responsible.
● Have check list of items attached to the trolley.
● Check that each item is:
– present;
– clean;
– working properly.
● Wash trolley daily.

Special equipment

Have detailed instructions of care written out both in the procedure book and close to the piece of equipment. Here is an example.

Ambu suction pump
This can be *life saving* if it is kept in good working order. It will *not* work if tubes are blocked.

When not in use
● Keep covered.
● Test every morning by sucking water, then empty the bottle and suck air through.

When in use constantly
Every day
● Remove stopper. Wash in soapy water.
● Rinse by holding *upside down* under running tap – to flush ball valve.
● Wash and rinse bottle. Attach drainage tube to outlet at top of bellows.
● Suck *soapy water* or *detergent* through *whole* apparatus.
● Suck *clean water* through.
● Suck *air* through.

Disinfection
● A disinfectant not harmful to the parts must be used, e.g. Savlon.
● Bottle and catheter can be boiled.
● Bellows can be cleaned by unscrewing the bolt under the base plate.
● Air outlet valve in bellows is reached by removing 3 screws under cover plate.

Responsibilities
● Sister in charge or staff nurse assigned by her to demonstrate.
● Each new student in the ward is responsible to make sure it *has* been demonstrated to her, within the first 3 days.
● *Daily care.* Nurse in charge of treatment room. If used in the

afternoon or *night* it should be cleaned out immediately and not left in a dirty state.

Why?   Because it can be life saving *if it is working.*

Equipment made at the hospital

Keep a list of these things in the ward procedure book, for example:
● Splints – write down the measurements of the various sizes and how many you have of each.

It is helpful to keep more detailed notes of some items, e.g. Restrainers.

Responsibilities for care

● **Everyone** – Certain responsibilities: e.g. To see the floor is kept free of rubbish – to report when something is broken.
● **Some responsibilities go with assignments** – e.g. If you are in charge of the treatment room, then you are responsible to see that all the trays such as mouth trays, are complete and clean. This does not mean you have to clean them all yourself. The suction pump and croupaire would also be in this category.
● **Some responsibilities go with procedures** – e.g. If you *use* the mouth tray then you see to it that everything is cleaned and returned to it. Alternatively, the procedure may be to set your own tray for use and clear away after use.
● **Some seem to belong to no one** – These have to be listed, and alongside the list, those who will care for maintenance.

Replacing and obtaining equipment

What about things we should have but have not got? If the staff were aware of the equipment they *should* have, and if they *kept on* asking for them until they got them, then children would suffer less. If a surgeon demands a scalpel and forceps, he will inevitably get them because they are considered essential to his work. Paediatric staff are sometimes hesitant in persisting in asking for what is equally vital for their work, for example, weighing scales and feeding tubes.

It may help to accelerate the process of obtaining equipment if you **keep a list of equipment and where it can be obtained**.

The quality of care is usually better when the medical and nursing staff have access to books and other learning material. A small reading room where the hospital staff can usefully spend a couple of hours every week refreshing their knowledge can become a valuable part of the hospital.

A number of useful texts and teaching slides may be obtained at low cost from the charity Teaching Aids At Low Cost (TALC). A great deal of thought and effort goes into the preparation of the texts and other teaching materials, which are all specifically prepared for health workers in the developing world. Currently TALC distributes 70 books and 60 sets of teaching slides. In addition 10 sets of slides on Primary Child Care are also available. Details of TALC list of books and slides may be obtained by writing to:

Teaching Aids At Low Cost,
P.O.Box 49,
St. Albans,
Herts AL1 4AX,
United Kingdom.

Some useful drug dosages

Aspirin   Tab. 300 mg and paediatric 75 mg.
  Give orally 4−6 hourly.
  Under 1 year use paracetamol.
  1−5 years 75−150 mg.
  6 years + 300 mg.

Aminophylline   in status asthmaticus.
  I.V. 4 mg/kg over 20 minutes.

Bephenium   Sachets 5 g.
  Under 6 years 2.5 g   Give fasting and
  7 years+   5.0 g.   no food for 1 hour.
                        Repeat in 1−2 days.

Choral hydrate   B.P.C. 500 mg/5 ml. Paediatric Elixir 200 mg/5 ml.
  Dose: 30−50 mg/kg up to maximum single dose of 1 g orally.

Chloroquine   Tab. 150 mg base.

Age/years	Up to 1 year	1−2	3−5	6−12
Initial	1/2	1	1	2
In 6 hours	1/2	3/4	1	1
Day 2−5 (daily)	1/2		1/2	1/2	1

I.M. if acutely ill − initial dose 5 mg/kg − then continue oral
  regime.

Chlorpromazine   Do not give under 2 weeks of age.
  Dose 1 mg/kg oral or I.M. 3−4/day.

Diazepam   Dose 8 or 12 hourly for sedation.
  Age   2/52 − 1 year   1 year   7 years
         250 microg/kg   1 mg   5 mg

Digoxin   Oral or I.M. Dose 1 or 2/day.
  10 microg/kg/day. No need for digitalisation.
  If required I.V. dose is half the stated dose.

Ephedrine   Elixir 15 mg/5 ml (in wheezing and asthma).
  Dose: 2 years 15 mg: 7 years 30 mg.

Ferrous sulphate   Tab. Ferrous sulphate Co. 220 mg. Paed. Mixture
  60 mg/5 ml.
  Dose: 15 mg/kg/day in 3 doses from age of 2 weeks.

Folic acid   Tabs. 100 microg, 500 microg and 5 mg.
  Dose once daily-orally.
  Up to 1 year 250 microg/kg − 1−5 years 2.5 mg − 6−12 years
  5 mg.

Frusemide   Dose: 1−3 mg/kg by mouth daily or on alternate days. I.M. half oral dose. I.V. quarter oral dose.

Hydralazine   Dose: From 1 year onwards 0.2 mg/kg/day in 4 divided doses. Maximum 200 mg/day oral or I.V.

Iron dextran (Imferon)   Ampoule 2 ml or 5 ml containing 50 mg iron/ml.
Haemoglobin above 6g/dl
Wt. in kg × 2/3 = total number mls iron dextran needed.
Haemoglobin below 6g/dl
Wt in kg = total number of mls iron dextran needed.
Give by deep I.M. injection in 0.5 − 1 ml doses until total dose given.

Levallorphan   Dose: 0.25 mg I.M. or I.V.

Levamisole (Ketrax)   Tab. 40 mg. Dose: 1−4 years 1 tab.
5−15 years 2 tabs.

Metronidazole (Flagyl)   Tab. 200 mg. Use only after 2 weeks of age.
Giardiasis 40 mg/kg (max. 2g) once daily for 3 days.
Amoebiasis 20 mg/kg (max. 800 mg) 3 times daily for 5 days.

Mepacrine   For giardiasis − Tab. 100 mg. Give 2/day for 5 days.
Under 12 kg − 25 mg. 12−20 kg − 50 mg. Over 20 kg − 100 mg.

Niridazole (Ambilhar)   Dose: 25 mg/kg/day orally in 2 doses for 5 days. Maximum single dose 500 mg.

Paraldehyde   Deep I.M. injection. Divide doses if more than 5 ml.
0.1 ml/kg up to 1 year. Then additional 1 ml/year up to 5 years to a maximum of 10 ml.

Rethidine   Dose 1 mg/kg oral or I.M. up to 3/day.

Phenobarbitone   To prevent spasms or fits: 3 − 6 mg/kg/day orally in 3 divided doses.
To treat fits: Birth to 1 year 6 mg/kg/dose by I.M. injection.
At 1 year − 30−60 mg I.M.
At 7 − 14 years 60 − 90 mg I.M.
For treating fits, diazepam or paraldehyde is better.

Phenytoin   Tab. 50 mg. Suspension 30 mg/5 ml.
Dose: 2−5 mg/kg twice daily orally.

Piperazine   Tab. 500 mg. Mixture 500 mg/5 ml.
Threadworms: 50 mg/kg once daily for 7 days.
Ascariasis: 100 mg/kg one single dose in the morning.

Propranolol   Avoid in neonates − then 1 mg/kg up to 40 mg orally 2−3 times a day.

Promethazine (Phenergan)   Dose: 1.5 mg/kg up to 25 mg at 7 years − orally 3/day.

Pyrantel   Dose: 10 mg/kg to a maximum of 1 g orally.

Theophylline for apnoeic attacks in neonates − 2 mg/kg 8 hourly orally.

Thiabendazol Dose: 50 mg/kg/day. Give orally in two divided doses a day for 3 days.

Antimicrobials

Note Drugs used in the treatment of Tuberculosis are in Chapter 10.

Ampicillin Neonates − 30 mg/kg I.M./I.V. 12 hourly.

Over 4 weeks − 50 mg/kg/day in 4 divided doses.

High dose − 200 mg/kg/day in 4 divided doses.

Ampiclox Neonatal suspension − 0.6 ml 4 hourly orally.

Injection − Ampicillin 50 mg/Cloxacillin 25 mg 8 hourly I.M./I.V.

Chloramphenicol Neonates 12.5 mg/kg/dose 12 hourly I.V.

4 weeks to 1 year − 12.5 mg/kg/dose 8 hourly I.V.

Over 1 year − 50 mg/kg/day orally in 4 divided doses.

Co-trimoxazole (Septrin) Tab. 480 mg. Give 12 hourly.

Dose: 6 weeks − 5 months 1/4 tab.

6 months − 5 years 1/2 tab.

6 − 12 years 1 tab.

I.M. injection − not under 6 years.

7 years + 3 mg/kg 12 hourly. Max. 160 mg single dose.

Erythromycin Oral − 50 mg/kg/day in 4 divided doses.

Injection − I.V. preferable to I.M. Dose 2.5 mg/kg 8 hourly.

Gentamycin Dose 2.5 mg/kg I.M. or I.V. 8 hourly.

If less than 7 days old give 12 hourly.

Penicillin G (Benzyl) Neonates − 25 mg/kg 8 hourly I.M./I.V.

4 weeks to 1 year − 15 mg/kg I.M. 6 hourly.

Severe infections 25 − 50 mg/kg I.V. over at least 5 minutes.

Triplopen Dose: 2 weeks − 1 year $\frac{1}{4}$ vial.

1 − 7 years $\frac{1}{2}$ vial.

7 − 14 years 1 vial.

Every 2 − 3 days I.M. only.

Streptomycin Neonates − avoid.

Dose: Over 4 weeks 25 mg/kg I.M. once daily to 7 years 500 mg daily and 1 g at 14 years I.M. once/day.

Sulfadimidine Neonates − avoid.

4 weeks − 1 year 25 mg/kg/dose 4 times a day.

At 1 year 250 mg and at 7 years 500 mg 4 times a day orally.

Trimethroprim Tab. 100 mg. Give 2/day.

Neonates avoid.

4 weeks − 1 year 4 mg/kg/dose.

At 1 year 50 mg and 7 years 100 mg/dose.

Abbreviations

ACTH	Adrenocorticotrophic hormone
APH	Antepartum haemorrhage
ASOT	Antistroprolysin 'o' titre
ATS	Anti-tetanus serum
b.d.	Twice daily
BP	Blood pressure
CNS	Central nervous system
CSF	Cerebrospinal fluid
DPT	Diphtheria, pertussis, tetanus vaccine
EBM	Expressed breast milk
ESR	Erythrocyte sedimentation rate
FG	French gauge
Hgb	Haemoglobin
IM	Intramuscular
INH	Isonicotinic acid hydrazide
i.u.	International units
IV	Intravenous
IVP	Intravenous pyelogram
LBW	Low birth weight
NG	Nasogastric
OPD	Outpatients department
ORS	Oral rehydration salt (solution)
PA	Per abdomen (refers to abdominal examination)
PAS	Para-aminosalicylic acid
PCV	Packed cell volume
PEM	Protein energy malnutrition
POP	Plaster of Paris
PPD	Purified protein derivative
PUO	Pyrexia of unknown origin
RC	Rural clinic
SS	Sickle cell
Tab	Tablet
TB	Tuberculosis
URI	Upper respiratory infection
VDRL	Veneral disease research laboratory test
wbc	White cell count
WF	White fluid

Index

344